CHOOSING DISINFECTION ALTERNATIVES FOR WATER/WASTEWATER TREATMENT

HOW TO ORDER THIS BOOK

BY PHONE: 800-233-9936 or 717-291-5609, 8AM–5PM Eastern Time

BY FAX: 717-295-4538

BY MAIL: Order Department
Technomic Publishing Company, Inc.
851 New Holland Avenue, Box 3535
Lancaster, PA 17604, U.S.A.

BY CREDIT CARD: American Express, VISA, MasterCard

BY WWW SITE: http://www.techpub.com

Choosing Disinfection Alternatives for Water/Wastewater Treatment

Frank R. Spellman, Ph.D.

TECHNOMIC PUBLISHING CO., INC.
LANCASTER · BASEL

Choosing Disinfection Alternatives for Water/Wastewater Treatment
a**TECHNOMIC**® publication

Technomic Publishing Company, Inc.
851 New Holland Avenue, Box 3535
Lancaster, Pennsylvania 17604 U.S.A.

Printed in the United States of America
10 9 8 7 6 5 4 3 2 1

Main entry under title:
Choosing Disinfection Alternatives for Water/Wastewater Treatment

A Technomic Publishing Company book
Bibliography: p.
Includes index p. 127

Library of Congress Catalog Card No. 99-62529
ISBN No. 1-56676-757-1

To George Armstrong Custer Redden
and Hugh Latham Bates

Table of Contents

Preface

SEVERAL years ago, G. C. White[1] (arguably the guru of chlorination) stated, "Just as water is close to being a universal solvent, so chlorine is nearly a universal water treatment chemical" (p. 256).

We can take White's statement a step further. "Just as water is close to being a universal solvent, so chlorine is nearly a universal water—and wastewater—treatment chemical." This modified statement reflects chlorine's actual use in water and wastewater treatment. Simply stated, chlorine has been the workhorse used in disinfecting both water and wastewater since the early 1900s, to the extent that when we speak on the topic, we typically refer to water/wastewater disinfection as *chlorination*—using it as a substitute term for the term disinfection. Remember, the primary objective of water/wastewater chlorination is disinfection.

Note that although we treat the terms *disinfection* and *chlorination* as if they are interchangeable (almost synonymous), chlorine has been found to serve other useful purposes in water/wastewater treatment. These uses include taste and odor control, prevention of algal growths, clean filter media maintenance, removal of iron and manganese, destruction of hydrogen sulfide, color removal by bleaching of certain organic colors, maintenance of distribution system water quality by controlling slime growths, restoration and preservation of pipeline capacity, restoration of well capacity, main sterilization, control of organisms responsible for bulking and foaming, and improved coagulation by activated silica.

Although some purposes of disinfection listed above apply to both water and wastewater, note that the primary objectives of wastewater disinfection are somewhat different from those purposes of disinfecting potable water. The primary objectives of wastewater disinfection are to prevent the spread of disease and to protect potable water supplies, bathing beaches, receiving waters used for recreational sports, and shellfish growing areas. The impor-

[1]G. C. White. *Handbook of Chlorination* (2nd ed.). New York: Van Nostrand Reinhold, 1986.

tance of chlorination disinfection also includes an important useful feature that, according to G. C. White, is often overlooked: wastewater disinfection has the useful ability to serve as a monitor for the combined wastewater treatment processes. "If all the unit processes are not performing properly the chlorination system will not be able to deliver an effluent that meets the NPDES discharge requirement" (p. 476).

At this point, the question becomes: So what? I know all this. What else is new? The answer to this question is what this text is all about. Another question is: What do you mean, this text is about what is new?

The following are reasons we are looking for something new for disinfection.

Are you familiar with OSHA's Process Safety Management (PSM), 29 CFR 1910.119, or USEPA's Risk Management Program or Plan (RMP), Section 112(r) of the Clean Air Act and 40 CFR Part 60? If you are presently using chlorine (Cl_2) or chlorine dioxide (ClO_2) to disinfect water or wastewater, and sulfur dioxide (SO_2) to dechlorinate wastewater (and other chemicals such as ammonia, both aqueous and anhydrous, or are producing digester biogas, and/or other listed hazardous substances), then you should already know all about PSM and RMP. If you are not aware of these two relatively new rules/regulations and their far-reaching requirements, then this text should definitely be required reading.

Another new consideration is important. On December 3, 1998, President Clinton announced new federal drinking water standards aimed at filtering out impurities and helping communities to upgrade their treatment systems. More effective and efficient filtration systems (already available commercially) will reduce dependence on chemical disinfection. These regulatory standards (The Disinfectant/Disinfection By-Product Rule (D/DBP) and the Interim Enhanced Surface Water Treatment Rule) are meant to simultaneously reduce health threats from bacteria and viruses and from the disinfectants used to remove them. They toughen standards for allowable concentrations of chlorine by-products in drinking water, regulate *Cryptosporidium,* tighten standards for turbidity from 5 to 1, and are estimated to reduce individual exposure to by-products, including trihalomethanes (THMs), by an estimated 25%. Municipalities already examining disinfection alternatives now have even more reason to put an alternative process into place.

For the moment, we will assume that you are familiar with PSM and RMP and that you are already in compliance with PSM (the deadline for compliance with OSHA's PSM requirement was May 27, 1997). Because USEPA's RMP compliance deadline is no later than June 21, 1999, we will assume that the affected reader is well on the way toward full compliance. We are making a lot of assumptions (and disregarding what they usually say about the term *assume*), but we are already in compliance. We know how important this subject matter is.

If you are familiar with PSM and RMP, you are also aware of the herculean task compliance presents for those who use listed chemicals, including chlorine and chlorine dioxide.

Simply stated, if you wish to continue using chlorine and other related chemicals for disinfection (or for any other treatment process), you must also implement strategies for compliance with two new rules that are somewhat costly and difficult to implement and to maintain.

One way to comply is to sidestep the issue entirely. But how? This question leads to several more. Are alternatives available? Are chemicals or physical processes available for disinfection that preclude the necessity for and the requirement to comply with PSM and RMP? The simple answer is yes. The compound answer is yes—to a degree.

This text is about these alternatives—about disinfection alternatives—about avoiding compliance with tricky and difficult regulations. Another important question people in responsible charge in water and wastewater treatment are asking is: If OSHA and USEPA have instituted tough regulations on the use of chlorine and other listed chemicals, and if we are in full and complete compliance with these regulations, is that enough?

This question haunts many of those in responsible charge in water and wastewater treatment. Because new regulations mandate communications over many different areas and conditions for the covered chemicals, will not this new regulatory push also work to alert the public—the politicians—the doomsayers—the lawyers? We think it will.

We must ask ourselves this question: Can we afford to continue to use chlorine and other covered chemicals in the normal operation of water and wastewater treatment operations without constantly worrying about liability? Only the responsible person in charge of such affected facilities can answer this question.

In this text, we present a treatment of typical disinfection techniques using chlorine (the workhorse of the industry), and the alternatives presently available for substituting chlorine with other chemical processes.

Presented in jargon-free plain English, *Choosing Disinfection Alternatives for Water/Wastewater Treatment* is designed to provide the reader with a description and discussion of alternatives to chlorine use for disinfection and other purposes. Although this text recommends substitution of other chemicals for chlorine to avoid costly, time-consuming compliance with the regulators, and to avoid possible litigation liability for chemical spills, keep in mind that substituting chlorine for other chemicals or physical processes is no pie-in-the-sky solution. For example, the costs of substituting chlorine with sodium hypochlorite will increase your operating costs approximately three fold.

FRANK R. SPELLMAN
Virginia Beach, Virginia

Acknowledgements

SPECIAL thanks to Joanne Drinan for graphic support.

CHAPTER 1

Disinfecting Water/Wastewater: What's It All About?

If you visit American city,
You will find it very pretty.
Just one thing of which you must beware:
Don't drink the water . . .(Tom Lehrer, 1965)

1.1 INTRODUCTION

HE wandered the foggy, filthy, corpse-ridden streets of 1854 London searching, making notes, always looking . . . seeking a murdering villain—and find the miscreant, he did. He took action; he removed the handle from a water pump. And, fortunately for untold thousands of lives, his was the correct action—the lifesaving action.

He was a detective, of sorts. No, not Sherlock Holmes but absolutely as clever, as skillful, as knowledgeable, as intuitive—and definitely as driven. His real name: John Snow. His middle name? Common Sense. Snow's master criminal, his target—a mindless, conscienceless, brutal killer: cholera.

Let's take a closer look at this medical super sleuth and at his quarry, the deadly killer cholera—and at Doctor Snow's actions to contain the spread of cholera. More to the point, let's look at Dr. Snow's subsequent impact on disinfection of both potable water sources and wastewater.

1.1.1 DR. JOHN SNOW

An unassuming and creative London obstetrician, Dr. John Snow (1813–1858) achieved prominence in the mid-nineteenth century for proving his theory (in his *On the Mode of Communication of Cholera*) that cholera is a contagious disease caused by a "poison" that reproduces in the human body and is found in the vomitus and stools of patients with cholera. He theorized that the main (though not the only) means of transmission was water contaminated with this poison. His theory was not held in high regard at first, because a commonly held and popular countertheory stated that diseases are transmitted by inhalation of vapors. Many theories of cholera's cause were expounded. In the beginning, Snow's argument did not cause a great stir; it was only one of many hopeful theories proposed during a time when cholera was causing great distress. Eventually, Snow was able to prove his theory. We describe how Snow accomplished this later (see Section 1.1.3), but for now, let's take a look at Snow's target: cholera.

1.1.2 CHOLERA

According to the U.S. Centers for Disease Control (CDC), cholera is an acute, diarrheal illness caused by infection of the intestine with the bacterium *Vibrio cholera*. The infection is often mild or without symptoms, but sometimes can be severe. Approximately 1 in 20 infected persons have severe disease symptoms characterized by profuse watery diarrhea, vomiting, and leg cramps. In these persons, rapid loss of body fluids leads to dehydration and shock. Without treatment, death can occur within hours.

Note: You don't need to be a rocket scientist to figure out just how deadly cholera was during the London cholera outbreak of 1854. Comparing the state of "medicine" at that time with ours is like comparing the speed potential of a horse and buggy to a state-of-the-art NASCAR race car today. Simply stated: cholera was the classic epidemic disease of the nineteenth century, as the plague had been for the fourteenth. Its defeat was a reflection of common sense, progress in medical knowledge, and of the enduring changes in European and American social thought.

How does a person contract cholera? Again, we refer to the CDC for our answer. A person may contract cholera (even today) by drinking water or eating food contaminated with the cholera bacterium. In an epidemic, the source of the contamination is usually feces of an infected person. The disease can spread rapidly in areas with inadequate treatment of sewage and drinking water. Disaster areas often pose special risks. As we write this, the aftermath of Hurricane Mitch in Central America is causing concern for a potential cholera epidemic.

Cholera bacteria also live in brackish river and coastal waters. Shellfish eaten raw have been a source of cholera; a few people in the United States have contracted cholera after eating raw shellfish from the Gulf of Mexico. The disease is not likely to spread directly from one person to another; therefore, casual contact with an infected person is not a risk for transmission of the disease.

1.1.3 FLASHBACK TO 1854 LONDON

The information provided in the preceding section was updated and provided by CDC in 1996. Basically, for our purposes, CDC confirms the fact that cholera is a waterborne disease. Today, we know quite a lot about cholera and its transmission, how to prevent infection, and how to treat it. But what did they know about cholera in the 1850s? Not much; however, one thing is certain: They knew cholera was a deadly killer. That was just about all they knew until Dr. John Snow proved his theory. Recall that Snow theorized that cholera is a contagious disease caused by a poison that reproduces in the human body and is found in the vomitus and stools of cholera victims. He also believed that the main means of transmission was water contaminated with this poison.

Dr. Snow's theory was correct, of course, as we know today. The question is, how did he prove his theory correct? The answer provides an account of one of the all-time legendary quests for answers in epidemiological research—and an interesting story.

Dr. Snow proved his theory in 1854, during yet another severe cholera epidemic in London. Although ignorant of the concept of bacteria carried in water, Snow traced an outbreak of cholera to a water pump located at an intersection of Cambridge and Broad Street (London).

How did he isolate this source to this particular pump? He accomplished this by mapping the location of deaths from cholera. His map indicated that most of the deaths occurred within 250 yards of that water pump (see Figure 1.1). The water pump was used regularly by most of the area residents. Those who did not use the pump remained healthy. Suspecting the Broad Street pump as the plague's source, Snow had the water pump handle removed and ended the cholera epidemic.

Sounds like a rather simple solution, doesn't it? For us, it is simple, but remember, in that era, aspirin had not yet been formulated—to say nothing of other medical miracles we take for granted, for example, antibiotics. Dr. John Snow, by the methodical process of elimination and linkage (Sherlock Holmes would have been impressed—and he was), proved his point, his theory. Specifically, through painstaking documentation of cholera cases and correlation of the comparative incidence of cholera among subscribers to the city's two water companies, Snow showed that cholera occurred much more frequently in customers of the water company that drew its water from the lower Thames, where the river had become contaminated with London sewage. The other company obtained water from the upper Thames. Snow tracked and pinpointed the Broad Street pump's water source. You guessed it: the contaminated lower Thames, of course.

Dr. Snow the obstetrician became the first effective practitioner of scientific epidemiology. His creative use of logic, common sense, and scientific information enabled him to solve a major medical mystery—to discern the means by which cholera was transmitted.

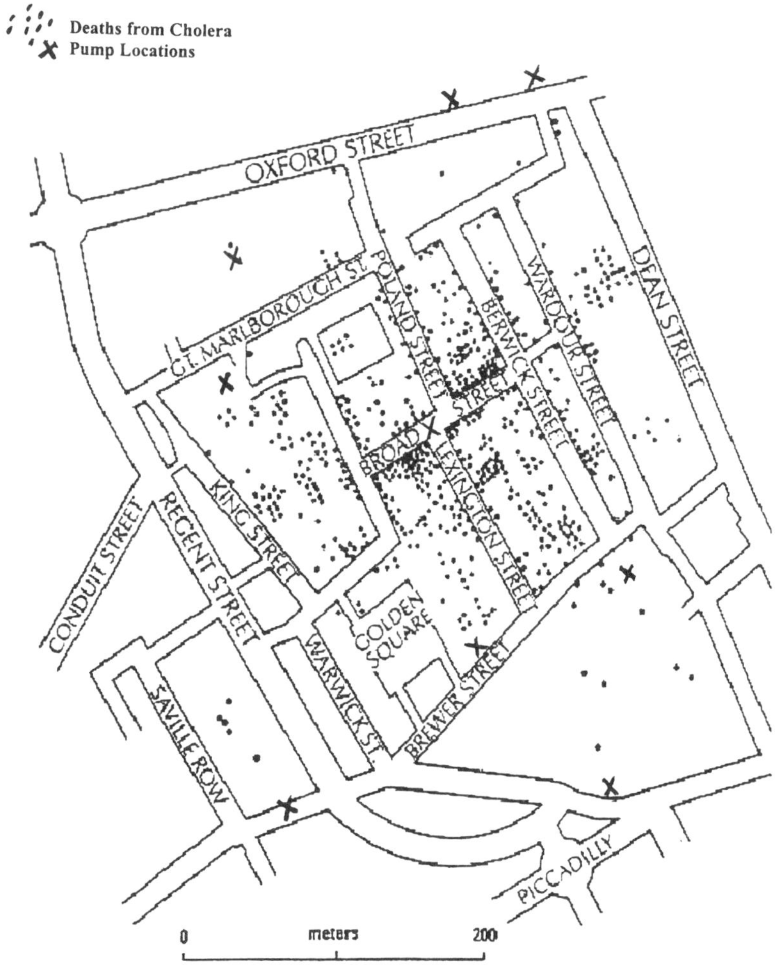

Figure 1.1 Dr. John Snow's map of cholera deaths and pump locations.

1.2 PUMP HANDLE REMOVAL—TO DISINFECTION

Dr. John Snow's major contribution to the medical profession,[2] to society, and to humanity in general can be summarized rather succinctly: He determined and proved that the deadly disease cholera is a waterborne disease.

What does all of this have to do with disinfection and with disinfection alternatives? Actually, Dr. Snow's discovery—his stripping of a mystery to its barest bones—has a lot to do with water and wastewater treatment

[2]Dr. John Snow's second famous medical accomplishment was that he was the first person to administer anesthesia during childbirth.

disinfection and disinfection alternatives. Combatting any disease is rather difficult without a determination of how the disease is transmitted—how it travels from carrier to receiver. Dr. Snow established this connection, and from his work and the work of others, progress was made in understanding and combatting many different waterborne diseases.

Today, sanitation problems in developed countries (those with the luxury of adequate financial and technical resources) deal more with the consequences that arise from inadequate commercial food preparation and the results of bacteria becoming resistant to disinfection techniques and antibiotics. We simply flush our toilets to rid ourselves of unwanted wastes and turn on our taps to take in high-quality drinking water supplies, from which we've all but eliminated cholera and epidemic diarrheal diseases. This is generally the case in most developed countries today, but it certainly wasn't true in Dr. Snow's time.

The progress in water treatment from that notable day in 1854 (when Snow made the "connection"—actually the "disconnection" of handle from pump—between deadly cholera and its means of transmission) to the present reads like a chronology of discovery leading to our modern disinfection practices. This makes sense, of course, because with the passage of time, pivotal events and discoveries occur—events that have a profound effect on how we live today. Let's take a look at a few elements of the important chronological progression that evolved from the simple removal of a pump handle to the advanced disinfection methods we use today to treat our water supply and our wastewater.

After Snow's discovery (that cholera is a waterborne disease emanating primarily from human waste), events began to drive the water/wastewater disinfection process. In 1859, 4 years after Snow's discovery, the British Parliament was suspended during the summer because the stench coming from the Thames was unbearable. According to one account, the river began to "seethe and ferment under a burning sun." As was the case in many cities at this time, storm sewers carried a combination of storm water, sewage, street debris, and other wastes to the nearest body of water. In the 1890s, Hamburg, Germany, suffered a cholera epidemic. Detailed studies by Koch tied the outbreak to the contaminated water supply. In response to the epidemic, Hamburg was among the first cities to use chlorine as part of a wastewater treatment regimen. About the same time, the town of Brewster, New York, became the first U.S. city to disinfect its treated wastewater. Chlorination of drinking water was used on a temporary basis in 1896, and its first known continuous uses for water supply disinfection occurred in Lincoln, England, and Chicago, Illinois, in 1905. Jersey City, New Jersey, became one of the first routine users of chlorine in 1908.

Time marched on, and with it came an increased realization of the need to disinfect both water supplies and wastewater. Between 1910 and 1915, technological improvements in gaseous and then solution feed of chlorine made the process more practical and efficient. Disinfection of water supplies and chlorination of treated wastewater for odor control increased over the next several decades. In the United States, disinfection, in one form or another, is now being used by more than 15,000 of approximately 16,000 Publicly Owned Treatment Works (POTWs). The significance of this number becomes apparent when you consider that fewer than 25 of the 600+ POTWs in the United States in 1910 were using disinfectants.

1.2.1 KEY DISINFECTION TERMS

A few pertinent terms relate to disinfection in general. Terms not included here are defined as they appear in the text.

- *disinfect* to inactivate virtually all recognized pathogenic microorganisms, but not necessarily all microbial life (cf. pasteurize or sterilize).
- *disinfectant* (1) any oxidant (including but not limited to chlorine, chlorine dioxide, chloramine, and ozone) added to water in any part of the treatment or distribution process that is intended to kill or inactivate pathogenic microorganisms; (2) a chemical or physical process that kills pathogenic organisms in water. Chlorine is often used to disinfect sewage treatment effluent, water supplies, wells, and swimming pools.
- *disinfectant time* the time it takes water to move from one point of disinfectant application (or the previous point of residual disinfectant measurement) to a point before or at the point where the residual disinfectant is measured.
- *disinfectant contact time* (T *in* CT *calculation*) the time in minutes that it takes for water to move from the point of disinfectant application or the previous point of disinfectant residual measurement to a point before or at the point where residual disinfectant concentration (*C*) is measured. Where only one *C* is measured, *T* is the time in minutes that it takes for water to move from the point of disinfectant application to a point before or where residual disinfectant concentration (*C*) is measured. Where more than one *C* is measured, *T* is:
  (1) For the first measurement of *C*, the time in minutes that it takes for water to move from the first or only point of disinfectant application to a point before or at the point where the first *C* is measured.
  (2) For subsequent measurements of *C*, the time in minutes that it takes for water to move from the previous *C* measurement point to the *C* measurement point for which the particular *T* is being calculated.

- *disinfection* a process that inactivates pathogenic organisms in water by chemical oxidants or equivalent agents.
- *disinfection by-products* compounds formed by the reaction of a disinfectant such as chlorine with organic material in the water supply.
- *waterborne disease* illnesses caused by pathogenic organisms in water/wastewater. The more common waterborne diseases are summarized in Table 1.1.

Note: Do not confuse disinfection with sterilization. *Sterilization* is the destruction of *all* microorganisms. Sterilizing potable water requires the application of a much higher dose of chemical disinfectants, which would greatly increase operating costs and would create taste problems for the consumer. Excessive application of disinfectants also generates excessive levels of unwanted disinfection by-products. Because of these problems, present treatment practices are used for turbidity removal and subsequent disinfection to the extent necessary to eliminate known disease-causing organisms sufficient to protect public health.

- *presence/absence of coliforms* presence of coliform bacteria in water is an indication that the water may be contaminated by pathogenic organisms. Absence of coliform bacteria is considered to be sufficient evidence that pathogens are absent if the source is good, a chlorine residual level is maintained, and the supply has a good history.
- *desirable characteristics of a disinfectant*
  (1) Must act in a reasonable length of time
  (2) Must act as temperature or pH changes
  (3) Must be nontoxic

TABLE 1.1. Major Waterborne Diseases.

Poliomyelitis
Meningitis
Hemorrhagic conjunctivitis
Hepatitis
Gastroenteritis
Typhoid fever
Bacillary dysentery
Cholera
Pneumonia
Tuberculosis
Giardia
Meningoencephalitis
Chronic anemia
Schistosomiasis

(4) Must not add unpleasant taste or odor
(5) Must be readily available
(6) Must be safe and easy to handle and apply
(7) Must be easy to determine proper concentrations
(8) Must be able to provide residual protection
(9) Pathogenic organisms must be more sensitive to disinfectant than are nonpathogens
(10) Must be capable of being applied continually
(11) Amount applied must be sufficient to produce a safe water

- *possible disinfectants*
  (1) Heat or boiling
  (2) Oxidizing agents—chlorine, ozone, bromine, iodine, potassium permanganate
  (3) Metal ions–silver, copper, mercury
  (4) Alkalis and acids
  (5) Ultraviolet light
  (6) pH adjustment to under 3.0 or over 11.0
- *deactivation mechanisms* (see Figure 1.2)
  (1) Damage the cell wall
  (2) Alter the ability to pass food and waste through the cell membrane
  (3) Alter the cell protoplasm

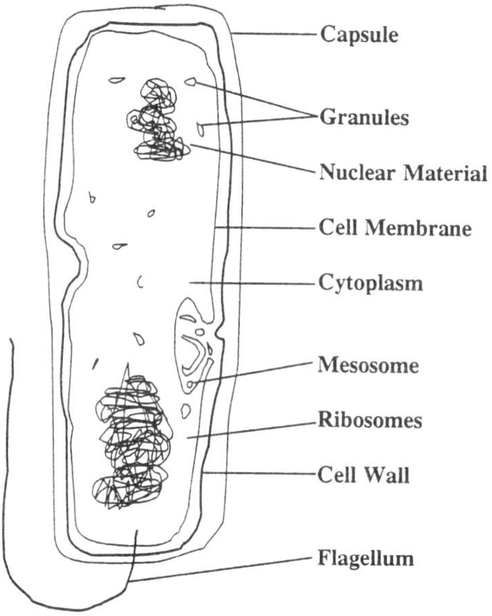

Figure 1.2 Bacterial cell.

(4) Inhibit the cell's conversion of food to energy
(5) Inhibit reproduction

- *importance of disinfection of water supplies* at the turn of the century, 35,000 of 1,000,000 people did not reach 20 years of age. Today, according to *USA TODAY* (1998) every minute, for every 101 deaths, there are 261 births. Curbing waterborne disease through disinfection has significantly contributed to births outpacing deaths worldwide.

1.3 ROLE OF DISINFECTANTS

Since the late 1970s, disinfection of water/wastewater has increased—disinfection has become more common (though not universally required by all states, nor even for all POTWs within a state). The impetus for the disinfection of wastewater effluents was provided by USEPA in 1972. Because of health risk concerns, in 1970, the EPA adopted a limit for coliform bacteria as part of its definition of secondary treatment.

USEPA did not mandate, however, disinfection of wastewater effluents without considering certain concerns. For example, biologists expressed concerns about the impact of chlorinated effluent on the receiving water ecosystems, specifically, the impact of residual chlorine on stream biota, especially fish. To address these concerns (and others), USEPA formed a task force to make recommendations on when disinfection was necessary, and how to minimize potential adverse impacts. The recommendations included:

- Disinfection should not be required where significant benefits are not proved.
- Prospective benefits of disinfection should be weighed against the environmental risks and costs.
- Chlorine should be considered only to control public health hazards.
- Chlorine should not be used where the protection of aquatic life is the primary consideration.
- Alternative means of disinfection or dechlorination must be considered where public health and aquatic life effects conflict.

The review of disinfection practices was also driven by the finding that chlorinated drinking water formed potentially carcinogenic halogenated carbon compounds. Although the concern applies to wastewater as well, exposure (at least to humans) is not direct. The more direct concern remains the acute toxicity of chlorine to biota in receiving streams. Recognition of the negative impact (at least in part) in 1976 led USEPA to rescind coliform concentrations as part of the definition of secondary treatment. In short, the major source of acute toxicity in POTW effluent (and thus, the chief environmental concern) is residual chlorine.

1.4 CHOOSING THE DISINFECTION ALTERNATIVE

To this point, we've mentioned few of chlorination's drawbacks in the disinfection of water and wastewater (potential carcinogenicity of certain compounds in water and damage to receiving stream's biota). That disinfection processes themselves can create hazards to human health and the aquatic environment is an obvious consideration, one that must be factored into the equation for determining and choosing the type of disinfection process to use at each individual plant—or whether to disinfect at all. In any case, the decision, either way, is at best a complicated one. As difficult as the disinfection selection process has been in the recent past, and as even more recent (1992) regulatory mandates regarding certain hazardous materials used in water, wastewater treatment, and other industries come on line, the decision becomes even more difficult.

When OSHA implemented its Process Safety Management (PSM) Standard (1910.119), and later when USEPA adapted OSHA's PSM into its own Risk Management Program (RMP) for accidental chemical release prevention under 112(r) of the Clean Air Act Amendments of 1990 covering facilities that handle explosive, flammable, or toxic (e.g., chlorine, ammonia, sulfur dioxide, and digester gas) materials above threshold quantities, the two organizations literally threw a monkey wrench into the equation.

With the aftermath of the Bhopal, India, incident and its tragic consequences and with chemical incidents closer to home, such as a spill in Institute, West Virginia, however, arguing against the need for OSHA's PSM and EPA's RMP rules would be difficult.

Note: Many facilities have already had to meet many of the RMP requirements under prior OSHA PSM requirements in effect since 1992.

In our experience over the past few years, we see that although costs are incurred for its development, a well-designed PSM/RMP program has the benefits of improved incident prevention and community and employee relations. We have also noticed improved operating performance and efficiency as a result of better training and safer operations. More importantly, implementation of these programs has contributed to fewer—and to avoiding altogether—catastrophic accidents, and to increased environmental protection. Industry as a whole is learning this, and those facilities required to comply with RMP will no doubt experience similar benefits.

But compliance with RMP is not problem-free. The problem? Actually, the problem is multifaceted. What does this mean? The answer is somewhat complex and lengthy to explain. However, we sum up the "problem(s)" associated with complying with RMP (specifically for water/wastewater operations, but also applicable to other covered industries) in Example 1.1.

Example 1.1

In our example we assume the following about the newly proposed Rachel's Creek Wastewater Treatment Plant (WWTP), which is still in the preconstruction planning stage. Because Rachel's Creek WWTP is still in the planning stage, some of the final decisions on its ultimate configuration and the chemical processes to be used are still being studied. One area under the scrutiny of design engineers (and especially of the customer—the owners and operators of the plant) is what type of disinfection will work best, taking into consideration RMP regulatory and other, nonregulatory, considerations. Look at some of the regulatory implications if the plant decides to install a chlorination/dechlorination system using elemental chlorine and sulfur dioxide to dechlorinate, and including other related chemical systems.

Initial considerations/specifications:

(1) Designed to treat 50 MGD
(2) Disinfection effected using elemental chlorine
(3) Dechlorination effected using sulfur dioxide
(4) Anhydrous ammonia used to provide nutrient feed
(5) Aqueous ammonia used for various treatment applications within various unit processes

OSHA PSM and EPA RMP thresholds for these chemicals are shown in Table 1.2.

For our purposes, let's assume that the plant exceeds the threshold limits for all four chemicals listed in Table 1.2. In a nutshell, this means that the proposed Rachel's Creek Treatment facility (and your facility, if it uses any of these covered chemicals and carries an inventory greater than the above thresholds) *must* comply with the following EPA Risk Management Program requirements:

- registration with EPA
- development and implementation of a comprehensive RMP

TABLE 1.2. PSM/RMP Thresholds.

Chemical	OSHA PSM Threshold	EPA RMP Threshold
Chlorine	1,500 lb	2,500 lb
Sulfur dioxide	1,000 lb	5,000 lb
Ammonia (anhydrous)	10,000 lb	10,000 lb
Ammonia (aqueous)	15,000 lb @ 44%	20,000 lb @ ≥20%

- submittal of an RMP to a central point yet to be designated by EPA with access provided to the implementing agency, State Emergency Response Council/Commission, Local Emergency Planning Committee, and the public

The EPA rule requires that a facility RMP be developed and implemented and an RMP Plan be submitted by June 21, 1999.

Exactly what would this mean for the Rachel's Creek wastewater treatment plant? What would they have to do to meet specific RMP requirements? RMP defines the following three major program components for the proposed Rachel's Creek treatment plant and for other facilities using or producing extremely dangerous substances:

- hazard assessment
- prevention program
- emergency response program

Note: EPA also established three tiers of requirements to reduce the level of effort for facilities with lower risk of off-site impacts, labeled Programs 1, 2, and 3. Program 1, for "no impact" facilities, has the fewest requirements, whereas Program 3 has the most (we assume for our example that Rachel's Creek meets the Program 3 requirement). Each facility will first have to complete several Hazard Assessment tasks and then determine which program is applicable, as described in Figure 1.3.

In Figure 1.3, *public receptor* means off-site residences; institutions; industrial, commercial, and office buildings; and parks or recreational areas inhabited or occupied by the public at any time without restriction. *Environmental receptor* means natural areas such as national or state parks, forests, or monuments; officially designated wildlife sanctuaries, preserves, refuges, or areas; and federal wilderness areas, which can be identified on local U.S. Geological Survey maps. WIPs are SIC Code 4941.

Program 1 "no impact" facilities must demonstrate that the worst-case release has no off-site consequences and that no accidents (chemical spill/release) have occurred in the last 5 years that caused off-site injury, death, or environmental degradation that required restoration actions.

1.4.1 RMP MAJOR PROGRAM COMPONENTS

1.4.1.1 Hazard Assessment

RMP requires a hazard assessment that includes evaluation of a range of releases (including worst-case accidental releases); analyses of potential off-site consequences; and a 5-year accident history. The hazard assessment must examine a range of accidental release scenarios, select a worst-case

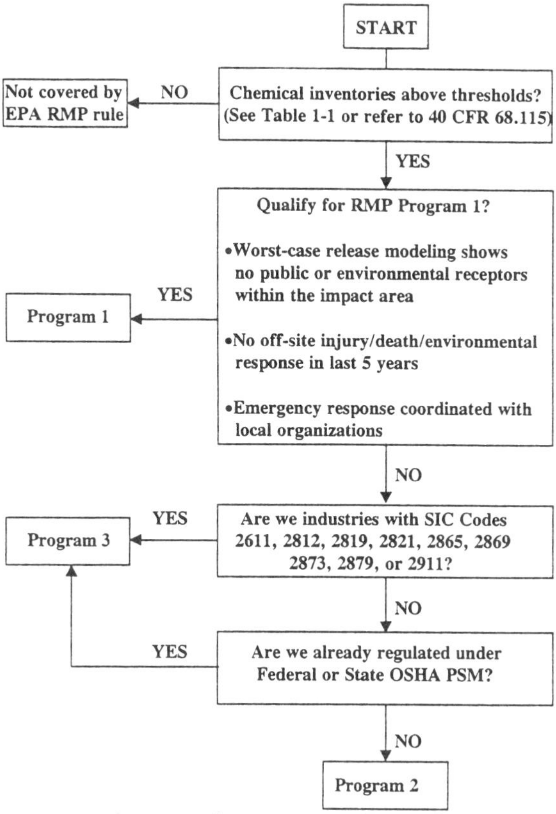

Figure 1.3 Applicability of EPA RM program rules and program classifications. *Source:* Adaptation from Puglionesi, P. S. (1998), p. 8.

accidental release scenario, analyze off-site consequences for the selected release scenarios including worst case, and document a 5-year history of significant accidental releases and accidental releases with the potential for off-site consequences. A hazard assessment must be completed for each regulated substance present above the threshold quantity. Facilities that use the regulated substance above its threshold in several locations or processes must evaluate a range of accidental releases and determine a worst-case release scenario for each location. The range of releases need only include those events that could lead to significant releases (i.e., accidental releases that have the potential to cause off-site death, injury, or serious adverse effects to human health or the environment).

Note: The definition of the worst-case scenario has been perhaps the most controversial aspect of the rule and one that could have a significant effect on public perception and emergency planning. The assumptions required for the worst-case release depend on whether the chemical is gaseous or liquid at ambient conditions, whether it is normally refrigerated, and whether it is listed due to toxicity or flammability.

For liquefied gases, the worst-case scenario is usually the release as a gas of the contents of the largest vessel over a 10-minute period. The EPA recognizes that the worst-case scenario may represent a highly improbable scenario—one that may not be the most appropriate for emergency planning. Because the results of worst-case scenario impacts can raise concerns, active communication efforts may be necessary to explain why basing emergency management plans and response capabilities on the worst-case may not be appropriate.

In addition to the worst-case release scenarios, the EPA requires facilities to analyze (if applicable) alternative release scenarios. RMP specifies several possible accident causes that facilities should consider when defining these "more likely" release scenarios. The list, however, should not be viewed as all inclusive. Each facility should examine its process to determine the event or sequence of events that may lead to significant accidental releases. When examining these potential release scenarios, facilities are allowed to assume that passive mitigation systems, such as containment dikes, function properly. Active mitigation systems, such as excess flow valves, fail-safe systems, scrubbers, flares, deluge systems, and water curtains, are assumed to fail.

The final element of the hazard assessment specified by RMP is a 5-year history of releases of covered substances. EPA interprets the accident history requirement to cover significant accidental releases and incidents that had the potential for off-site consequences, because CAA section 112(r) is directed at preventing such releases. Specifically, EPA requires the accident history to document releases that caused—or had the potential to cause—off-site consequences. The history must include the substance and quantity released, the concentration of the substance when released, and the duration of the release; the date of the release, time of the release, and any off-site consequences (e.g., evacuations, injuries, and environmental effects) must also be included.

1.4.1.2 Prevention Program

The Prevention Program covers safety precautions and maintenance, monitoring, and employee training measures. Since we stated that the proposed Rachel's Creek treatment plant will be a Program 3 plant, Table 1.3 lists the RMP Prevention Program requirements for Rachel's Creek and for other Program 3 entities.

Those familiar with OSHA's PSM may notice that RMP's Program 3 prevention program includes most of the PSM elements. Remember, both

TABLE 1.3. RMP Prevention Program Requirements.

Prevention Program 3 40 CFR 68.65–.87
Management system
Process safety information
Process hazard analysis
Operating procedures
Training
Mechanical integrity
Management of change
Prestart-up review
Compliance audits
Incident investigation
Employee participation plan
Hot work permit
Contractors

the OSHA PSM and EPA RMP rules emphasize the application of performance-oriented management programs rather than the application of specific requirements. The following sums up the key compliance points for Program 3.

Management: Because all of the prevention program elements must be integrated into a management system that is implemented on an ongoing basis, EPA requires that the owner or operator of the facility designate a single person or position as responsible for the development and implementation of the overall program. At facilities where individual elements of the program are handled by different people or divisions, the names or positions of the people responsible for each element are to be specified, and an organization chart or similar document is required to define the lines of authority. The purpose of the management requirement is to have facility management define a system that integrates the implementation of the elements and assigns responsibility for that implementation.

Note: On the basis of our experience, facilities that implement this element without strong management structure (and the backing of upper management) find the task to be difficult, if not impossible.

Employee participation: Employers must develop a written plan describing how they will involve employees in hazard analysis and other PSM elements, and how they will provide employees access to all PSM information.

Process safety information: The required process hazard analysis (see below) must be based on up-to-date chemical and process information, including information on physical and chemical hazards, process technology (e.g., process chemistry and process parameters), and equipment (e.g., equipment specifications and design and piping and instrumentation diagrams). All required process safety information applies only to affected equipment, not to the facility as a whole. Chemical information is available from Material Safety Data Sheets (MSDS) mandated under OSHA's Hazard Communication Standard (29 CFR 1910.1200). The level of process technology and equipment information varies with the type of facility.

Process hazard analysis: In the AIChE's *Guidelines for Hazard Evaluation Procedures* (AIChE, 1992), a hazard evaluation (a process hazard analysis) is defined as a procedure intended to identify the hazards that exist, the consequences that may occur as a result of the hazards, the likelihood that events may occur as a result of the hazards, the likelihood that events may take place that would cause an accident with such a consequence, and the likelihood that safety systems, mitigating systems, and emergency alarms and evacuation plans would function properly and eliminate or reduce the consequences.

What this all means is that a process hazard analysis must be performed (i.e., Checklist, What If Analysis, HAZOPs, and FMEA). This hazard analysis must be revalidated and updated once every five years, and the two most recent analyses must be retained on active file.

Operating procedures: From the results of the process hazard analysis, from information developed during the design of the process, and from industry and facility experience, a standard set of operating procedures must be developed for each covered process. Basically, the operating procedures describe the tasks to be performed by the operator, the operating parameters (e.g., temperature and pressure) that must be maintained, and the safety precautions needed for both operations and maintenance activities. Operating procedures must specify the consequences of deviations from safe operating limits (e.g., if the safe operating temperatures are between 120 and 160°C, the operating procedures should indicate what happens if the temperature is above or below those limits). Written operating procedures (they must be in writing) provide a guide to safe operations in a form that can be used by employees. Lack of operating procedures and inadequate operating procedures have been implicated in a number of catastrophic accidents. Operating procedures for covered processes must include instructions on steps for each operating phase (i.e., initial start-up, normal operation, emergency shutdowns, normal shutdowns, and emergency operations), operating limits, safety and health considerations, and safety systems. The facility must provide for control of hazards during operations involving lockout/tagout, confined space entry, and opening process equipment or lines, and have written operations procedures that specify entrance control to the facility by support personnel.

Training: Training provides employees with the information needed to understand what they must do to operate safely and why safe operations are necessary. The required training program is the key to ensuring the effectiveness of other program elements, such as operating procedures, maintenance programs, prestart-up reviews, and emergency response. All employees involved in working with covered processes must be thoroughly trained in process and safety (including emergency) procedures. Training consists of initial, refresher, and supplementary training. The employer must document that each employee has received the required training.

Caution: You can accomplish all the training required, provide the best training possible, hire the best trainers available, train the smartest employees in the world, but one thing is certain: If you do not document the training, then according to EPA/OSHA, your training did not occur. Both EPA/OSHA and the legal system will certainly take this view.

Contractors: Employers must ensure that contractors working near these processes are informed of all hazards related to the work and the emergency action plan. Employers must evaluate safety performance before contractor selection (e.g., review the contractor's OSHA 200 Log), log contractor injury and illness, and periodically evaluate contractor performance.

Prestart-up safety review: Start-up of a new or modified system can be a particularly hazardous time for facilities, especially for complex processes and those that require high temperatures, high pressures, or potentially exothermic reactions. RMP-covered facilities must ensure safety before a procedure goes on-line by reviewing procedures and checking all critical systems prior to start-up of a new or substantially modified process. This review includes a list of items that operators need to check or test before beginning an operation.

Note: Because all process installations will be "new" for Rachel's Creek personnel, this will demand special consideration. A prestart-up safety review is not only required, it is critical for maintaining a safe workplace and protecting the community from off-site consequences for catastrophic release of covered chemicals.

Mechanical integrity: Under RMP, the prevention program must include requirements for equipment maintenance. Preventive maintenance, inspection, and testing of equipment are critical to safe operations at the facility. Waiting for equipment to fail is not an acceptable approach, especially considering the extremely hazardous characteristics of the regulated substances.

Hot work permit: An authorization and permit program for welding, brazing, and grinding activities near or around these processes must be implemented and maintained by the employer or his representative.

Management of change: Remember that chemical processes are integrated systems; changes in one part of the process can have unintended effects in other parts of the system. For example, installation of better rupture disks may increase the pressure in vessels. Thus all changes in processes, chemicals, and procedures must be reviewed prior to their implementation, to identify any potential hazards that may be created by the modification. Although true that most changes at facilities are intended to improve safety and efficiency, any modification can have unintended effects and requires a specific review of the safety implications of the change.

Incident investigation: Accidents can provide valuable information about hazards and the steps needed to prevent accidental releases. Since Rachel's Creek Treatment Plant is still on the drawing board, it has not yet experienced any chemical accidents, obviously. However, for those Program 3 plants that are on line, this element requires that when chemical accidents do occur, they are investigated. Incident investigation, reporting, and documentation procedures must be prepared and implemented for any incident that did or could have resulted in an emergency situation. When Rachel's Creek plant goes on line, these procedures must be in place and ready for immediate use.

Compliance audits: In-house compliance audits must be performed at least once every three years to verify that the program elements are in place and that they have been implemented effectively.

Trade secrets: Only OSHA PSM explicitly states that secrets must be made available to employees if needed to meet PSM responsibilities.

1.4.1.3 Emergency Response Program

Both PSM and RMP specify that the emergency response program must include actions to be taken to protect human health and the environment in response to a release. These actions include informing the public and local agencies, planning for emergency health care, and employee training. Emergency response procedures are a necessary part of a risk management program, because accidents do happen, even with the best safety programs and systems in place. Emergency response procedures can reduce the severity of a release and protect employees, emergency responders, and the public from harmful exposure to the regulated substances.

Each facility must develop an emergency response plan that defines the steps the facility and each employee must take during an accidental release of a regulated substance. The plan must include both evacuation or protective action procedures for employees not directly involved in the response to the release, and the action taken by employees responsible for responding to and mitigating the release. All employees are to be trained in applicable emergency response procedures. The emergency response plan must include descriptions of all response and mitigation systems.

The emergency response plan must also include procedures for notifying the public of releases and of appropriate protective actions and procedures for notifying public agencies. The facility is required to develop information on proper first aid and emergency medical care necessary to treat accidental human exposure.

Note: Keep in mind that if a covered facility decides that its emergency response action(s) only requires the dialing of 911 and the evacuation of the plant site during a chemical emergency, the off-site responders must be familiar with the chemicals and processes used on the site and with the site itself. Do not assume that dialing 911 lifts the burden of responsibility and liability from plant management's shoulders. It does not. In a court of law, you could find yourself being held liable for the consequences of the spill. Remember, off-site emergency responders must become familiar with your plant site. This can only be assured by inviting them onto the plant site and walking them around it, pointing out the hazards as you tour the plant and by repeating this procedure annually or when new equipment that might affect their performance comes on line.

1.4.2 IS RMP REALLY REQUIRED?

Seems like a logical question, doesn't it? Actually, it depends more on point of view than anything else. For example, the concerned public (especially those living right outside the Rachel's Creek plant and other similar plants) probably feel that RMP is required—a reasonable precaution for community protection. The affected parties—the affected facility owners/operators? They probably sum it up as just another regulatory hassle—an unwanted, unnecessary, costly regulation shoved down their throats by the Feds—the USEPA. We like to call it the "chlorine killer" because that's the common response to learning that RMP is required.

Whatever the view might be, RMP is the law of the land, and compliance for "covered" entities is mandatory (see Figure 1.3).

Having said what no one really wants to hear, we illustrate why the USEPA feels so strongly about implementing RMP at facilities that store, produce, and use extremely hazardous substances (listed substances). Because we have been talking about wastewater treatment (in particular, Rachel's Creek Treatment Plant), in Example 1.2 we illustrate our point using another wastewater treatment plant—one that uses chlorine for disinfection.

Example 1.2[3]

The last rays of the setting sun touched the running waters of the large river that courses its way through the downtown area of a large metropolitan area. A plant operator at the 100 MGD wastewater treatment plant, located in the city along the same river bank, was walking the plant site making her rounds. Stopping at a sample point, she pulled a sample and then deposited the sample and its bottle into the carrying tray. Grabbing the tray, she

[3]From F. R. Spellman's *A Guide to Compliance for PSM/RMP*. Lancaster, PA: Technomic Publishing Company, Inc., 1997, pp. 3–6.

proceeded down the long winding stairway from #8 secondary clarifier. At the foot of the stairs she stepped onto the gravel path and proceeded toward the final effluent sampling point.

She walked along the path and then turned to her right. Straight ahead, just behind the 55-ton chlorine rail tank car, she noticed a yellowish-reddish glow.

Recognizing the yellowish-reddish glow for the brush fire that it was, the operator dropped the sample tray and ran the 250 feet to the plant's main control center to alert the shift lead operator about the brush fire near the chlorine tank car. While she dialed 911, the lead operator activated the site emergency alarm and used his portable radio to direct a plant assistant operator to meet him at the tank car.

With the plant's emergency alarm wailing its penetrating shrill noise throughout the plant site and the neighborhood, the lead operator and assistant were standing together approximately 100 feet from the chlorine tank car. They could see the brush fire was growing in strength; it was being fed by a brisk wind.

The lead operator wondered what to do next; his mind was blank. Then it cleared and a series of instantaneous thoughts entered his mind. First, he understood the gravity of the situation: an intense fire was about to engulf 55 tons of chlorine. Second, he realized there was no way he and the assistant operator could move the tank car out of harm's way. Third, he realized the spur line the tank car was positioned on was heavily overgrown with brush (just 2 weeks earlier he had intended to cut this overgrowth, i.e., whenever he could find the time to do it). As the operator and assistant advanced a few yards closer to the tank car, the operator noticed another problem. A plant maintenance crew had stacked a pile of wooden cement forms next to the spur line, within a few feet of the car; these forms were on the same side of the car where the fire was quickly approaching. The operator knew he would have to act fast to prevent an extremely dangerous situation from becoming a major catastrophe.

He had to do something. He did. The lead operator directed the assistant to go over to the nearest building, the NPW (nonpotable water) pump house, and bring a fully charged fire hose back to the fire with him. Then the lead operator darted off in the opposite direction, toward the chemical handling building, to get another fire hose.

About 5 minutes later both operators, manning two fully charged 1.5-inch fire hoses, approached the tank car from the side opposite where the brush fire had already reached the spur and had ignited the wood cement forms; the fire was beginning to grow, to burn with purpose.

Standing to one side with his fire hose directed at the midsection of the chlorine tank car body while the assistant, at the other end of the tank car, began directing a steady stream of water in the same general area, the lead operator could feel the heat from the growing fire.

A few minutes later the fire was burning the entire stack of wood cement forms, generating such intense heat that both operators had to move back a few feet from the car. At that same moment the tank car emergency relief valve, having reached its design activation pressure, lifted, releasing a controlled stream of chlorine (gas) into the atmosphere.

The operators could hear the sirens of emergency response vehicles approaching the plant site. Then the emergency relief valve failed completely. Now, instead of releasing a controlled amount of chlorine gas, the entire contents of the tank were escaping full force—a steady stream of yellow-green toxic gas, all 55 tons.

About six-tenths of a mile away from the treatment plant and the fire, at about the time the emergency relief valve on the 55-ton chlorine tank car had failed, evening classes at the community college were in progress. The 400 college students had heard the plant site emergency siren and then the other sirens as emergency vehicles raced by the college campus toward the wastewater treatment plant, but they paid them no mind. They had heard these alarms several times before; emergencies in central city were a common occurrence.

Meanwhile, back at the plant, the operators were now fully engulfed by the chlorine's yellowish-green cloud of death; they were about to take their last breaths. In the plant control room the operator who had discovered the fire and sounded the alarm had been busy. Not only had she notified the authorities about the emergency at the plant, she had also called the plant manager and chief operator and filled them in about the fire.

When she heard the emergency responder's sirens, she ran outside just in time to see the fire department and local Hazardous Materials (HazMat) team enter the plant site through the front gates. However, because darkness had set in, she did not see the dense yellowish-green cloud of chlorine gas that she walked right into. Instantly overcome by the chlorine gas, she fell to her knees coughing and gasping for air. Instead of air, she filled her lungs with deadly chlorine gas; she died 5 minutes later.

The emergency responders were not familiar with the plant site they had entered; they had not been invited to tour the plant site to learn the layout of the site. However, from information provided to the 911 operator, the emergency responders did know about the fire and the 55-ton tank car of chlorine. From knowledge they had gained through their training, they understood the danger involved with chlorine gas and fire. What they did not know, however, was that the fire had already reached the chlorine tank car, that the tank car emergency relief valve had already activated, and had released its entire load into the atmosphere.

However, these firefighters and HazMat responders knew their jobs. They had been properly trained in hazardous materials emergency response procedures; therefore, as they entered the plant site they were cautious. They were also alert enough to recognize, with the help of their spotlights, that the yellowish-green cloud of death was moving toward them.

It didn't take long before the Fire Captain in charge of this emergency situation gave the order for his responders to retreat to safer ground; they did.

Meanwhile, at the community college, two blocks from the treatment plant—less than 600 feet away—class had ended and students poured out of their classrooms. Several students left the building to go home. Others stepped outside for a few minutes to smoke cigarettes.

About the time the emergency responders were exiting the plant site to set up a command post in a safe zone, the chlorine cloud, driven by the same brisk wind that had steered the fire toward the tank car was pushing the ground, hovering poisonous gas toward the front entrance of the college buildings where students were socializing.

Within a few minutes the chlorine cloud came face to face with the college students. Several of the students survived the chlorine gas with only minor respiratory irritation. A few were more seriously affected; they were rushed to a local hospital. An even smaller number of students, those in the parking lot fronting the school, were more profoundly affected; later, three of these students died.

During daylight the next day and for several days after this incident, investigators and other interested viewers had little trouble following the path the deadly chlorine cloud had taken. Its path was clearly marked by dead grass, flowers, insects, bushes, and trees.

The incident just related points to the purpose of OSHA's Process Safety Management Standard and EPA's Risk Management Program. Both of these regulations are designed to prevent and/or detail the proper mitigation procedures to be used during hazardous material incidents. PSM and RMP not only function to set requirements for *on-site* emergency response planning and training, they also point out the need for emergency response planning for *off-site* consequences.

To gain a better sense of the positive impact that compliance with PSM and RMP can have on facilities that use or produce covered chemicals in their processes, consider the previous disaster scenario from a different point of view. That is, the preceding tank car incident could have developed in a much different manner if the elements and procedures required by both PSM and RMP had been in place and had been followed.

In the first place, PSM and RMP require that all responsible parties survey their industrial complexes where covered chemical processes are used and to closely scrutinize these processes to determine if any of the 100+ Highly Hazardous Chemicals listed in OSHA's Process Safety Management Standard and/or if any of the 140 Extremely Hazardous Substances listed in EPA's Risk Management Program are stored, handled, used, or produced on site.

In the chlorine tank car scenario, compliance with PSM and RMP would have ensured that the wastewater treatment plant had been thoroughly surveyed for processes using or producing highly hazardous chemicals and extremely hazardous substances. This survey would have determined, of course, that the plant site used chlorine, a covered chemical, in its process. Moreover, the survey would have noted the normal quantity of chlorine stored on the plant site at any given time. This survey would also have made note of the fact that the quantities of chlorine stored on the plant site exceeded the PSM and RMP Threshold Quantities of 1,500 and 2,500 lb, respectively, for chlorine (chlorine stored on the plant site in quantities at or above the threshold quantities require the plant to meet all the mandatory compliance requirements required by PSM and RMP).

Along with a complete survey of covered chemicals under PSM and RMP, several other benefits would have been gained through full compliance. These additional benefits can be summed up simply. For example, to comply with PSM and RMP, the plant site would have been required to complete the following actions:

(1) Plant management would have been required to perform a Process Hazard Analysis (PHA) for the entire chlorine process. During this PHA, all other plant processes using or producing covered chemicals would have been audited and a determination would have been made as to whether these processes used or produced other Highly Hazardous Chemicals or Extremely Hazardous Substances. More importantly, "What if" scenarios would have been developed, to determine the consequences of a fire engulfing the chlorine tank car, and a determination made on how best to prevent such an occurrence.
(2) Because the plant used chlorine at levels greater than the threshold quantity level listed in Table 1.2, plant management would have been required to comply with all regulatory requirements as related in the regulations.
(3) One of the important elements of PSM and RMP regulations that the plant would have been required to comply with is on-site and off-site consequence analysis or modeling to assess potential on-site/off-site exposures.
(4) Another important PSM and RMP element is the requirement for emergency response planning. This emergency response planning is required for both on-site and off-site (public areas).
(5) Plant operator training in proper HazMat Response is also required by PSM and RMP. The plant operators who responded to the fire and then the chlorine leak would have been trained on how to properly handle this incident. This particular element is absolutely critical. How critical?

To answer this question, take another look at the fire and the chlorine incident again from a different view—a completely different view, the correct view.

Let us assume (disregarding the standard saying about this term) that the plant operators determine that the fire might cause the temperature and thus the internal pressure of the tank car to be raised to a dangerous level. With this increase in internal tank pressure, the tank car emergency pressure relief valve would lift and release chlorine to the environment. Under PSM and RMP the operators would have been properly trained to respond to this situation in a correct manner. For example, when they first responded to the fire, they knew that the other operator was notifying the proper authorities; thus, professional help would have been on its way in a matter of a few minutes. Moreover, they also knew that by using the cooling water from the fire hoses they might be able to cool the tank car to a level where the tank car could have been maintained to a safe temperature level. As a matter of fact, it was what they did not know that produced the massive cloud of deadly chlorine gas that killed them, the other victims, and sent the Fire Department and HazMat Team in retreat.

If the plant operators had been properly trained in HazMat emergency response procedures, in the case of 55-ton chlorine tank car emergencies, they would have known some basic facts about tank cars and chlorine gas that could have brought about a different result. For example, the operators would have been trained on how to properly cool a tank car involved in fire. If properly trained, they would have known that the 55-ton tank car was designed to withstand the effects of most fires, that is, chlorine tank cars must be constructed as specified by the U.S. Department of Transportation (USDOT). USDOT specifies that all chlorine tank cars are to be protected with 4 inches of insulation. Thus, when the operators were directing their fire hoses at the midsection of the tank car body, they were not only wasting their time but also cooling water; they were providing little protection for the tank car's most vulnerable device: its pressure safety valve (PSV). Because the tank car's most vulnerable spot is the top housing (dome area), where the car pressure safety valves are located, the lead operator should have directed his water at the dome area and the assistant operator should have used a nozzle that produced a fine wet mist spray to cover the lead operator and protect him against the heat of the fire. The plant operators should have known this basic, standard fire-fighting technique. However, as was clearly demonstrated by their actions, they did not. They did not know the proper response procedures because they had not been trained.

Another safety issue must be considered. Because the operators were responding to a fire that involved deadly chlorine gas, why were they not properly attired in required personal protective equipment (PPE)—where were their respirators, their SCBAs—and other appropriate PPE? We have to wonder if the responders had been properly attired in PPE, would they have not stood a better chance of surviving? We think they would have.

Note: This incident also points to a serious lack of management oversight concerning the tank car itself—the high brush and wood cement forms stacked along the tank car should obviously not have been there.

Proper compliance with PSM and RMP would have helped mitigate this incident, of this there can be little doubt. Moreover, proper compliance with PSM and RMP would have helped in another way (actually, in several other ways). For example, full compliance with these regulations would have ensured that the local fire department and HazMat team would have been familiar with the layout of the wastewater treatment plant and had full knowledge of the plant site's chemical hazards. Most importantly, prior to this incident, plant site operators and emergency responders would have been required to meet, discuss, and walk through contingencies such as the tank car fire. The purpose of having such a meeting and discussion is to determine the best method to use in combatting all possible chemical emergencies.

If this plant site had been in full compliance with PSM and RMP, the local community college administrators (as part of the regulations' requirements for the right of the public to know the chemical hazards they might be exposed to in the event of a plant emergency) would have understood the meaning of the shrill alarm that sounded at the plant site when the chlorine emergency first occurred. The college administrators would have had the knowledge they needed to properly react to the emergency and correctly evacuate the college.

As graphic and terrible as the example of the chlorine tank car incident just described is, it should be pointed out that hazardous materials incidents do not always result only because of fire. Along with the constant threat posed by fire there are also chemical disaster situations that can occur because of human error in system operation and/or a malfunction in system equipment. There are other emergency situations that must also be considered and planned for, including floods, hurricanes, earthquakes, tornadoes, snow/ice storms, avalanches, explosions, truck accidents, train derailments, airplane crashes, building collapses, riots, bomb threats, terrorism, and sabotage.

From the preceding list of emergency situations, it should be obvious that the occurrence of any of the events listed could lead to an emergency situation that might reach beyond the boundaries of any plant or industrial site. This is to be expected, especially in this age of population explosion with its characteristic sprawl. It is not unusual to find, for example, a water/wastewater treatment plant or other industrial plant that was once isolated from city dwellers and then later became surrounded on all sides by neighbors. The point is that when a chlorine spill occurs in an isolated area, there may be no cause for general alarm; however, when such a spill occurs in the plant site described, it should be clear that the purpose of Process Safety Management, Risk Management Program, and other safety-related factors is far-reaching—and lifesaving.

1.5 THE BOTTOM LINE

The planners, designers, owners, and operators of Rachel's Creek Wastewater Treatment Plant obviously need to factor in the requirements of OSHA's PSM and EPA's RMP when they determine which chemical disinfection process to install. From the information related above, we see the obvious costs associated with using chlorine, sulfur dioxide, and other covered chemicals. Are the costs within reason? Is the owner/operator (if the chlorine option is chosen) willing to accept the responsibility, the cost, and the burden of complying with PSM/RMP? These questions must be answered, but the answers are site and locality specific.

So, what did Rachel's Creek decide to do? What disinfection alternative did they select for installation in their new plant? Right now, the jury is still out; they haven't looked at the alternatives we discuss in this text, but they will. We will answer these questions and explain the Rachel's Creek decision later in the text (see Chapter 10).

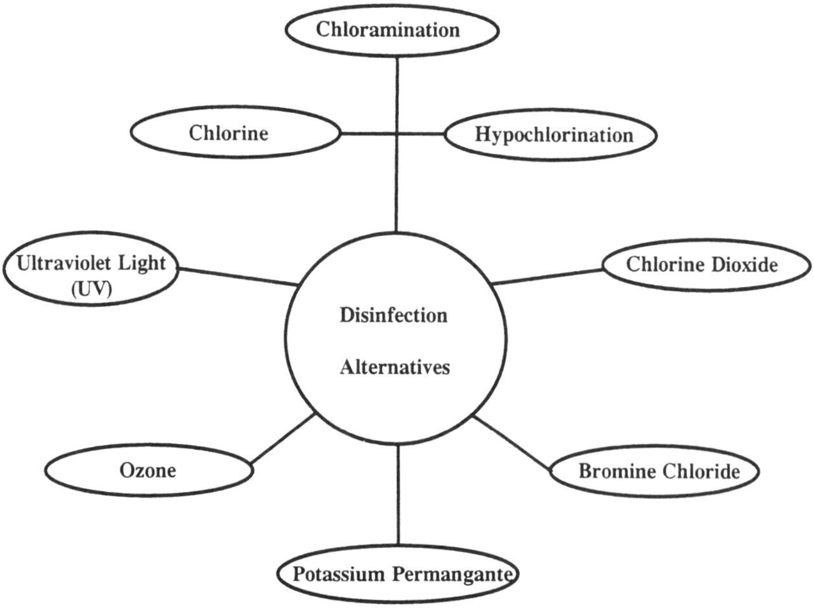

Figure 1.4 Disinfection alternatives.

TABLE 1.4. Major Factors in Evaluating Disinfectant Alternatives.

Effectiveness	Ability to achieve target levels of selected indicator organisms Broad spectrum disinfecting ability Reliability
Use-cost	Capital cost Amortization cost Operating and maintenance cost Cost of special wastewater pretreatment
Practicality	Ease of transport and storage, or ease of on-site generation Ease of application and control Flexibility Complexity Ability to predict results Safety considerations
Pilot studies required	Dose requirements Refine design details
Potential adverse effect	Toxicity to aquatic life Formation and transmission of undesirable bioaccumulating substances Formation and transmission of toxic, mutagenic, or carcinogenic substances

Rachel's Creek staff has a great deal of information to consider. For example, are there alternatives to chlorine use for disinfection in water, wastewater, and other applicable industries? The simple answer—yes, there are alternatives (see Figure 1.4). The compound answer?—yes, maybe there are, depending on site specific and local regulatory compliance requirements.

What does this compound answer really mean? It means that alternative chemical disinfection processes are available. We discuss them in this text. However, only the affected entity can make the determination as to whether the alternatives are suitable to meet their requirements in *all* respects.

In evaluating disinfectant alternatives (along with PSM/RMP requirements), many factors must be considered: the disinfectant's effectiveness, use-cost, practicality, pilot studies required, and potential adverse effects. USEPA (1986) lists and describes these evaluation factors (see Table 1.4).

Note: Keep in mind that no matter which factor or factors you consider on the way to making the ultimate decision on which disinfection alternative to use, the main consideration must be that the disinfection requirements (i.e., the need) should be evaluated on a case-by-case basis with consideration of beneficial use and criteria.

Other considerations that should be examined include ensuring that disinfection is used only when significant benefit can be derived from such use.

In all cases, the prospective disinfection benefits to be derived must be weighed against the environmental risks and costs. Chlorine should only be considered for use when public health hazards are present to control. Alternative disinfection methods and/or dechlorination must be considered when and where public and aquatic health and/or life impacts coexist.

No "generic" disinfection alternative or procedure exists; the Clean Water Act and site-specific criteria drive the selection process. This is the real bottom line.

1.6 DISINFECTION ALTERNATIVES: WHAT IS THE ANSWER?

In our Rachel's Creek wastewater treatment plant example, we illustrate some of the considerations that go into determining which disinfection alternative is "best" for the particular plant involved. Rachel's Creek treatment plant obviously has a huge advantage over many other active plants or industries. The advantage? Rachel's Creek is a new construction project. Isn't it always easier and more cost effective to install a particular system (any system) in new construction than it is to retrofit a facility that is already constructed and on-line? The simple answer: Yes, absolutely. New construction is easier and in most cases more cost-effective. The compound answer: Well, maybe, or maybe not; just as there is no "generic" disinfection alternative, there is no "generic" answer to this question. Remember, your decision must be driven by regulatory compliance requirements and site-specific criteria.

So, what is the answer? How can you choose the best disinfection alternative for your facility? Should you choose any alternative at all? That is, should you stay with what you have at present?

All of these questions are good ones, of course. Actually, these are the questions that drove the writing of this text. Why? Because we asked ourselves these same questions, and after a painstaking process, we answered them.

As stated earlier, in this text we provide you with an explanation of these answers (see Chapter 10). We explain what Rachel's Creek WWTP did and what disinfection alternative they ultimately chose and why. Think about this hint on what their final choice will be—a concern that drives them to their ultimate determination. They took into consideration the increasing need for wastewater treatment plant upgrading modifications, including more stringent disinfection criteria, elimination of design deficiencies, and expanding the state-of-the-art for process design. They considered the science, the pilot studies, and the results. They did all this and then they violated one cardinal rule: "Base decisions on sound science and not on just what feels good or right." They did what felt right and good for them. Was it the right decision? Only time will tell. One thing is certain; what felt good and right was driven by the (their) public—and the regulations, of course. Why? Simply put, when the neighbors and the regulators are happy, Rachel's Creek is happy. When the plant doesn't have to worry about regulators, they are actually ecstatic, delighted, delirious, elated, overjoyed—and greatly relieved. OK, let's hype it a bit: They were jumping with joy!

Do you know these feelings? Have you been there? If not, we highly recommend going there.

1.7 REFERENCES

AIChE. *Guidelines for Hazard Evaluation Procedures* (2nd ed.). New York: Center for Chemical Process Safety of the American Institute of Chemical Engineers, 1992.

Lehrer, T. *That Was the Year That Was.* Reprise Records R6179, 1965.

Puglionesi, P. S. *Preparing for EPA's New Risk Management Program (RMP) Regulations.* Haverton, PA: Duke Engineering and Services, Inc., 1998.

Spellman, F. R. *A Guide to Compliance for PSM/RMP.* Lancaster, PA: Technomic Publishing Company, Inc., 1997.

USA TODAY, October 1998.

USEPA, *Design Manual: Municipal Wastewater Disinfection.* Washington, DC: U.S. Government Printing Office, 1986.

1.8 SUGGESTED READING

Dennison, M. S. *OSHA and EPA: Process Safety Management Requirements.* New York: Van Nostrand Reinhold, 1994.

Isaac, R. A. Disinfection dialogue: the evolving perception of need, benefit and detriments. *Water Environ. Technol.,* 8, 5, 67–72, 1996.

Plumbing and Mechanical Engineer, *Pipeline*, 7, 3, summer 1996.

Spellman, F. R. *Confined Space Entry.* Lancaster, PA: Technomic Publishing Company, Inc., 1998.

Rosenburg, C. E. *The Cholera Years.* Chicago: The University of Chicago Press, 1987.

White, G. C. *Handbook of Chlorination* (2nd ed.). New York: Van Nostrand Reinhold, 1986.

CHAPTER 2

Elemental Chlorine

Pollution, Pollution.
They got smog and sewage and mud,
Turn on the tap and get hot and cold running crud. (Tom Lehrer, 1965)

NOTE: For simplicity and to demonstrate the efficacy (or lack of efficacy) of each disinfection alternative, in *Choosing Disinfection Alternatives for Water/Wastewater Treatment,* we focus on the process used to select an alternative disinfection process for a planned construction project. For this real-life process, the fictional facility we use is called Rachel's Creek Wastewater Treatment Plant. We could as easily have chosen a new construction water treatment plant to demonstrate the same process, but wastewater treatment is often more complex than water treatment, so we use it as the model in this text.

Note that the process of selecting the disinfection system for use at Rachel's Creek is just one methodology that may be used to make the selection. We chose the particular method described in the rest of this text for one simple reason: We have used it and it was effective.

Are better and more thorough methods available? Most assuredly. Did this method work for us? Yes.

The opinions stated here are the author's alone—the author's point of view and interpretation of the research materials, which means that there may be a better way and certainly a considerable difference of opinion. But we consider that a positive, open, informed discussion and shared information on these methods makes the selection process easier for all.

2.1 INTRODUCTION

The General Manager of the Sanitation Authority that owned and would operate the plant after its construction assigned the prospective managers and other key personnel for Rachel's Creek Wastewater Treatment Plant

(WWTP) the task of performing an evaluation of disinfection alternatives for the WWTP. After completing a thorough review of the alternatives, the team's written report was to be turned over to the Authority's General Manager (GM). The team's evaluation report was to include a recommendation on which disinfection alternative the team thought most suitable for use at Rachel's Creek WWTP. This final recommendation was to be submitted to the General Manager within 60 days of the convening date: after the report was submitted, the GM would make the ultimate, final decision on which disinfection process would be installed at Rachel's Creek.

The team was formally named the Disinfection Selection Team (or DST). The team leader, the chairperson (Nancy Jo), was selected by the General Manager from the Sanitation Authority's management core. She was directed to select six members to staff the team. From the prospective hires already chosen for Rachel's Creek facility, Nancy Jo selected the prospective plant manager, the chief operator, lead operator, maintenance chief, safety director, and from outside the Authority, she selected a licensed environmental engineer from a well-known and highly respected wastewater engineering firm.

The DST met for the first time in August of 1998. At this first meeting, Nancy Jo laid out the agenda—the plan of attack for selecting the proper disinfection system for Rachel's Creek WWTP.

Following the guidelines provided in USEPA's *Design Manual: Municipal Wastewater Disinfection* (1986) the team decided on the major factors to be considered in evaluating disinfection alternatives. The list of factors included:

- effectiveness
- use-cost
- practicality
- pilot studies required
- potential adverse effects
- regulatory requirements under PSM/RMP

Next, the chairperson stated that whichever disinfectant was chosen, Rachel's Creek had to meet or exceed *all* regulatory requirements (i.e., permit).

The chairperson also explained that the actual process to select the disinfection system might require two levels of review. In the first level of review, only the nonmonetary factors were to be considered. This qualitative assessment was comprised of three primary components, including technical factors, environmental impacts, and safety. To accomplish this, a qualitative matrix approach was to be used (see Table 2.1). After the selection process progressed from alternative to alternative, assessments would be ranked, to aid in making a final determination as to which alternative was best suited for Rachel's Creek and the Authority. Nancy Jo laid out a plan that would

TABLE 2.1. Disinfection Selection Team's (DSTs) Matrix for Determining the Applicability of Alternative Disinfection Techniques.

Alternative Disinfection Technique (e.g., Cl_2, BrCl, and O_3)
Consideration
Size of plant
Applicable level of treatment prior to disinfection
Equipment reliability
Process control
Relative complexity of technology
Safety concerns—transportation on-site
Bactericidal
Virucidal
Fish toxicity
Hazardous by-products
Persistent residual
Contact time
Contributes D.O.
Reacts with ammonia
Color removal
Increased dissolved solids
pH dependent
O & M sensitive
Corrosive
Covered by PSM/RMP*

*DST modification.
Source: USEPA, 1986.

include analyses to narrow the appropriate alternatives and completely eliminate (hopefully) some of the alternatives.

The plan was to take the alternatives left over from the initial screening process (assuming more than one alternative was left) and give them a more detailed evaluation. If a second level of review was required, a preliminary design should be developed, cost estimates performed, and an economic analysis comparing the alternatives on an equitable basis could then be evaluated. Detailed capital, operation, and maintenance costs would be developed for each alternative disinfection system.

The alternative disinfection systems to be reviewed included the following, presented in the order in which they are to be reviewed:

- elemental chlorine (see Figure 2.1)
- hypochlorination
- chloramination
- chlorine dioxide
- bromine chloride
- potassium permanganate

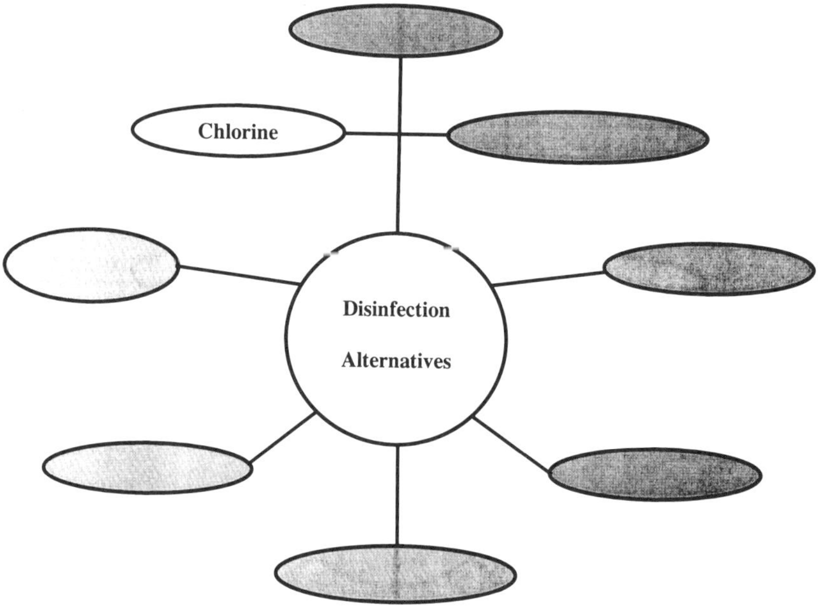

Figure 2.1 Chlorine alternative.

- ozone
- ultraviolet light (UV)

These disinfection alternatives are shown in Figure 1.4.

Before we describe the DST's disinfection technique evaluation process, let us point out that even before the DST met for the first time, a bias toward selecting elemental chlorine for Rachel's Creek WWTP existed for several reasons. The most important reason was the Authority's experience with using elemental chlorine at its nine other WWTPs, as well as its two Water Treatment Plants (WTPs). The Authority's GM told the chairperson, right up front, that she would be hard-pressed to change his mind about using anything but chlorine for disinfecting wastewater. She would have to put forward a strong recommendation and convincing evidence of the need to use any technology other than elemental chlorine before he would be convinced.

If the GM was already sold on using chlorine, then why study the alternatives at all? The chief reason? The GM had been informed by the Authority's Safety Director that chlorine was now a dinosaur (his opinion) for disinfecting water/wastewater.

The Safety Director explained his point of view, which revolved around the relatively new regulatory requirements of USEPA's Risk Management

Program (RMP). "Because of RMP, the EPA has virtually killed chlorine use in many industries," stated the Safety Director (his opinion, but one strongly supported by empirical evidence). Then the Safety Director went into a long-winded (but precise) description of RMP and its requirements. He stressed again and again the difficulties inherent in the requirement to let the public know about the chlorine, about the potential affects/effects of a catastrophic release of chlorine gas into the neighborhood surrounding the treatment plant, and all the other regulatory requirements. He also informed the GM that all pertinent information on listed chemicals—including chlorine—would have to be made available to the public on the internet.

The Safety Director's hyperbole (if that is what it was) planted a seed of concern in the GM's mind about the actual practicality of choosing the chlorine disinfection alternative for Rachel's Creek WWTP.

Thus, although not absolutely convinced to use anything else but the old industry workhorse chlorine, the GM was also smart enough to realize that a study of the alternatives was called for. Indeed, he not only wanted to see the pros and cons for each alternative technique but also he was determined to cover any decision he might make with documentation, with empirical data and with a good faith effort.

Why? Well, most of the reasons are quite obvious—sounds like a good management decision to me. Consider this; you've heard of the burr under the horse's saddle, the same one that eventually causes the rider to be thrown. A burr (RMP compliance) was now firmly planted under the GM's saddle. He didn't like the data he'd heard on RMP. Too many years of experience with following EPA and OSHA regulations allowed him to imagine what compliance to RMP would mean, and he was determined to remove the burr or to know the reason why it was still there. In the end, he did.

The chairperson was fully aware of the GM's bias toward chlorine use as the primary disinfectant of choice at the Authority. Nancy Jo felt significant amounts of pressure as chairperson: the person who would have to sign and present the final review—perhaps one that he would disagree with. She also knew that her team would have to deliver a report to the GM that he would be able to digest without any heartburn; if burn developed, it would certainly end up being transferred to her own gastrointestinal tract (and elsewhere). She was professional and no jelly fish. She had backbone. The moniker "smart" is an understatement in her case. She was smart enough to know that the GM would never have authorized the formation of the DST to look at disinfection alternatives for no reason at all.

In this chapter and the chapters to follow, we look at the methodology used and material the DST reviewed in selecting the best alternative disinfection technique for Rachel's Creek Treatment Plant. Chapter 10 presents the DST's recommendation and the reasoning behind it; we also state the choice the GM bought into—the choice that would remove the burr.

Take a closer look at the points the DST came up with and listed for review of the first disinfection alternative: elemental chlorine.

2.2 ELEMENTAL CHLORINE (Cl_2): SOME BASIC POINTS

The DST assigned the future Safety Director of Rachel's Creek the task of recorder for the team. Each item (bulleted below) found, mentioned, discussed, researched, or otherwise—the good, the bad, and the ugly—he listed on a series of flip charts for later study and review.

The team began the listing process:

- Disinfection of drinking water/wastewater is one of the main achievements of our time in the quest to protect the public health. The primary player in this accomplishment: chlorine.
- The use of chlorine for the destruction of microbiological pathogens has been essential in protecting the public from outbreaks of waterborne disease.
- Chlorine, as well as other disinfectants, produces a variety of chemical by-products.
- The risks from the presence of microbial pathogens in drinking water/wastewater effluent is estimated to be several magnitudes greater than the risk from chlorination by-products.
- Some water plants have rejected chlorine because the public didn't want chlorine and accused it of harboring carcinogens and of having a disagreeable smell and taste.
- The July 1998 *Chicago Daily Herald* reported: "Chlorine Exposure Sends 11 to Hospital." The report went on to state: ". . . chlorine that was a by-product of mixed chemicals was the culprit. The cloud dissipated very quickly . . . People came in this morning and complained about irritated throats." "No injury was considered life-threatening," firefighters said.
- Chlorine is a cost-effective way to kill bacteria, viruses, and other harmful substances found in water, whether from decaying leaves, from runoff, or from industrial pollution.
- Chlorine is a gas that's wondrously useful in protecting public health, except for one little problem: it can kill you (*The Commercial Appeal,* 1998).
- Faced with new federal regulations (PSM and RMP) and concerns about potential releases, many facilities throughout the country are having second thoughts about use of chlorine gas in disinfecting water/wastewater.
- Even though many facilities have a very good record with chlorine, it is a very dangerous substance.

- Under one section of the Clean Air Act, major users of chlorine and other chemicals that could cause catastrophic accidents in communities must draw up elaborate emergency-response plans.
- The chlorine in the water/wastewater is not dangerous to humans, because concentrations are maintained at a safe level.
- Despite decades of chlorine use, most facilities using chlorine have not experienced any significant release.
- Nationwide, dangerous releases of chlorine from water/wastewater plants are rare.
- Nonetheless, EPA's RMP rule will require (21, June 1999) facilities having at least 2,500 pounds of chlorine on site to conduct risk assessment planning and prepare contingency reports. This includes reviews of safety records and preparation of maps of release zones showing areas where dangerous concentrations of chlorine would drift in the event of a worst-case scenario.
- RMP also may require some chlorine handlers to install expensive scrubbing equipment capable of neutralizing any escaping gas.
- A 1-ton release of chlorine could spread a cloud of harmful concentration for more than 6 miles.
- In addition to the cost and paperwork burdens of RMP, many utilities worry about the public relations fallout from the worst-case scenario maps (which are to be made public).
- Because of the toxicity of chlorine residuals at extremely low concentrations, it is difficult to control chlorine-induced toxicity in the receiving stream. Therefore, use of alternative disinfection processes should be considered where adequate toxicity is the overriding concern (USEPA, 1986).
- The use of chlorine disinfection of wastewater can result in several adverse environmental impacts, especially from toxic levels of total residual chlorine in the receiving waters and the formation of potentially toxic halogenated organic compounds. Chlorine residuals have been found to be acutely toxic to some species of fish at very low levels. The chlorine residuals are stable and can persist for many hours at toxic levels. Other toxics or carcinogenic chlorinated compounds can bioaccumulate in aquatic life and contaminate public drinking water supplies (USEPA, 1986).
- Chlorine has been relatively safe to transport from shipper to receiver and throughout plant sites throughout the nation.
- Elemental chlorine systems are reliable and flexible, and the equipment is not complex. It is relatively easy to apply and control in wastewater treatment, and low use cost is often its greatest advantage. Even when dechlorination is required (as it is at Rachel's Creek), it is still the lowest cost alternative in most cases (USEPA, 1986)

- Besides its use to disinfect wastewater effluent, chlorine is commonly used in odor control in wastewater and foul air, prevention of septicity, control of activated sludge bulking, and cyanide destruction.
- Dechlorination can completely remove chlorine-induced toxicity.
- According to G. C. White (1986), the importance of chlorination disinfection also includes an often overlooked, but important, useful feature: wastewater disinfection has the ability to serve as a monitor for the combined wastewater treatment processes. "If all the unit processes are not performing properly the chlorination system will not be able to deliver an effluent that meets the NPDES discharge requirement" (p. 476).
- Chlorination for disinfection follows all other steps of treatment. The purpose of chlorination is to reduce the population of organisms in the wastewater to levels low enough to ensure that pathogenic organisms will not be present in sufficient quantities to cause disease when discharged.

After completing the initial list of chlorine concerns, the DST reviewed each item on the list and highlighted important points, prioritized them, and then moved on. The DST then reviewed basic information and facts about elemental chlorine itself.

2.2.1 BASIC ELEMENTAL CHLORINE INFORMATION

The Safety Director listed the following details and information about elemental chlorine on the flip charts from information gathered by the team for the team's review.

- Forms of chlorine:
  (1) Gas—compressed into a liquid, stored in steel containers
  (2) Solid—calcium hypochlorite; in tablet or granule form
  (3) Liquid—sodium hypochlorite solution; household bleach
- Selection criteria:
  (1) Amount of wastewater to be treated
  (2) Configuration of WWTP
  (3) Availability of the chemicals
- Terminology:
  Available chlorine can provide some disinfection if same amount of available chlorine is added; measurement of available chlorine in pounds; and dose—available chlorine fed
  Chlorine a strong oxidizing agent that has strong disinfecting capability

Chlorine concentration milligrams per liter (mg/L) or parts per million (ppm)
Chlorine residual remaining concentration after a specific time period at a given point
Chorine demand
(a) Demand = Dose – Residual
(b) mg/L, ppm, or lb
(c) Amount consumed

Chlorine contact time
(a) Time between addition and measurement point
(b) Fixed by pump rate and storage tank
(c) 30 minutes minimum

Chlorine residual
(a) Usually determined by testing
(b) 0.2 to 0.4 mg/L "free"
(c) Changes with time
(d) Protects against outside contamination and regrowth
(e) Collected:—before out falled—where and when bacteriological samples are taken

2.2.2 GAS CHLORINATION

- Stored in 100, 150, 2,000-lb pressurized containers; 55- and 90-ton railroad tank cars
- 99.9% pure; assume 100% pure, with each pound composed of only available chlorine
- Compressed liquid expands to a gas when released, requiring heat
- 2 gallons will fill a $4 \times 4 \times 8$ room (128 ft^3)
- 2.5 times heavier than air
- gas greenish-yellow in color
- gas seen at 100 ppm
- gas smelled at 3.5 ppm
- gas corrosive in moist air
- throat irritant at 15 ppm
- death at 1,000 ppm
- does not burn but supports combustion
- requires a separate, gas tight room with forced ventilation

2.2.3 SAFETY CONSIDERATIONS

- Feed and storage rooms must be isolated.

- Doors must open to outside with panic hardware.
- One air change per minute (acm) is required.
- Exhaust at floor level is required.
- Do not use exhaust fans with motor attached to the fan blades.
- Use negative ventilation.
- Place air inlet at ceiling.
- Place fan switch outside.
- Wear goggles, gloves, aprons, and full face shield.
- When changing containers/cylinders, SCBA is required.
- Gas detection system must be installed.
- Emergency response procedure is required.
- Full compliance at Program 3 Level for PSM/RMP is required.

2.2.4 FACTORS IMPORTANT TO SUCCESS OF CHLORINE (Cl_2) DISINFECTION

- concentration of chlorine
- contact time
- temperature of the wastewater
- pH of the wastewater
- TSS in the wastewater

2.2.5 TYPICAL CHLORINE (Cl_2) OPERATION: PROCESS DESCRIPTION

Note: Because the DST Chairperson wanted to ensure that the team covered all the bases for the use of elemental chlorine, she and her team decided that their study should include information regarding process operation of a chlorination system. For this reason, we provide an operational description of a typical chlorination system. The Safety Director (and the DST recorder) included the following information in the DST report. The system described takes feed from ton cylinders.

Chlorination: process description: Chlorine is a very reactive substance. Added to wastewater at levels to satisfy all chemical demands, it reacts with certain chemicals, such as sulfide, sulfite, and ferrous iron. The chlorine used by these reactions is chemically changed (reduced) and is no longer available for disinfection purposes. The chlorine used up in these reactions is known as chemical demand. Chlorine will also react with ammonia to produce chloramines (chemicals consisting of chlorine, nitrogen, and hydrogen; see Chapter 4).

Note: Chloramines are combined chlorine.

The chloramines have some disinfecting capability and show up in combined residual when performing a chlorine residual test. After all of the chemical demands are met, chlorine will react with water to form hypochlorous (HOCl) and hydrochloric (HCl) acids. The hypochlorous acid (HOCl) is the most effective form of chlorine for disinfection and is known as free residual. In most wastewater treatment plants, the chemicals present in the wastes make trying to achieve a free residual impractical. For this reason, wastewater disinfection is usually accomplished using the combined residual. The process is controlled by monitoring the total residual chlorine (TRC). For most domestic wastes, disinfection requires chlorine concentration of μ 1.0 mg/L for at least 30 minutes at design flow. To ensure actual detention time is close to the calculated hydraulic detention time, most chlorine contact tanks are usually designed with baffling to prevent short-circuiting. Contact tanks normally are designed to provide a tank length to width ratio of μ 20:1 and a depth to width ratio of 1:1 (see Figure 2.2).

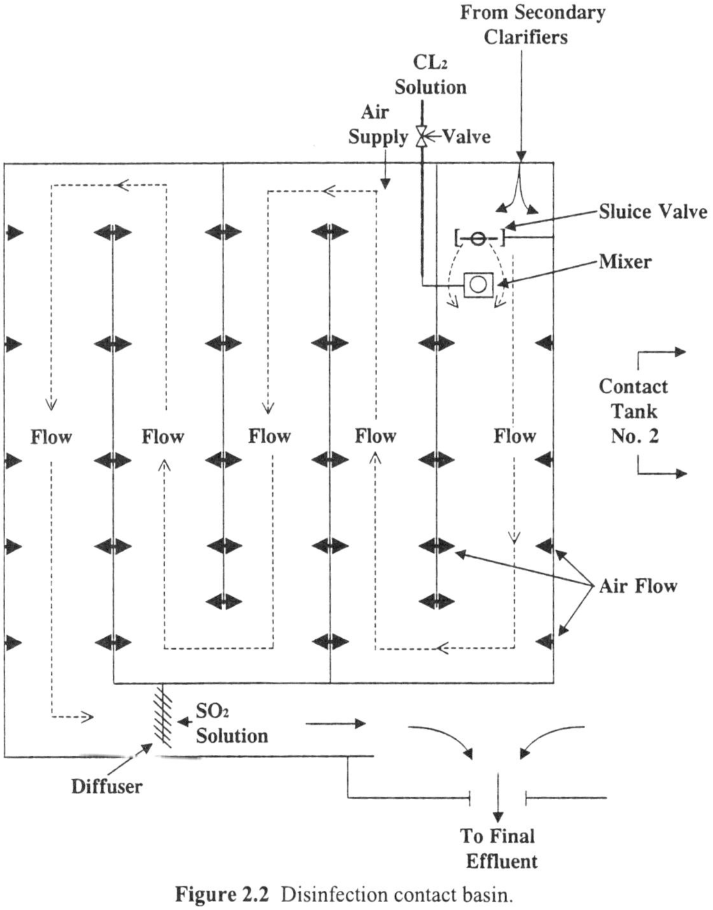

Figure 2.2 Disinfection contact basin.

The DST decided the chlorination process description provided to this point was good, but not good enough. According to the chairperson, what they really wanted to study and to later reference (if need be) was an actual unit process operation. She also recalled the GM's statement: ". . . you will be hard-pressed to change my mind about using anything but chlorine for disinfecting wastewater at the Authority." Yes, Nancy Jo recalled these words; in fact, she had written them down at the top of her massive notepad. She liked to stay in focus, and her focus was on what the GM had told her. Thus, she convinced the DST that they all needed to have a basic understanding of the chlorine disinfection process—how it actually operates, especially at the Authority. "You never know when we are going to have to stand before the 'big man' (the GM) and have to explain in detail how our decisions were made . . . and there is one thing for certain, I *will* know something about the chlorine disinfection process!" Thus, the DST sought additional information on the elemental chlorine disinfection process and included this material in the notes that follow.

Because the Authority's other wastewater and water treatment facilities already used elemental chlorine in ton containers, they decided to include a unit process operational description in the report. Although somewhat detailed in nature, the next section covers the unit process description from the DST's report.

2.2.6 UNIT PROCESS OPERATION (ACTUAL)

The disinfection unit process consists of the following system at the Authority's water/wastewater treatment plants:

- chemical feeding
- contact tank

The purpose of disinfection is to destroy pathogenic (disease-causing) organisms in the wastewater, a process accomplished by adding chlorine (a toxic chemical) to the wastewater flow and holding the flow for the appropriate amount of time to effect an essentially complete kill. The contact (or holding) tank (see Figure 2.2) is designed so that little mixing occurs within the tank. This ensures that all the wastewater is held for the appropriate time period. A residual amount of chlorine after the appropriate time period indicates that a suitable amount of disinfectant has been added. At Authority plants, chlorination is followed by dechlorination using sulfur dioxide (like chlorine, an RMP-covered chemical). The final effluent is dechlorinated to remove any residual chlorine before disposal. Disinfected flow is typically disposed of or reused.

2.2.6.1 Disinfection Chemical Feeding

The purpose of disinfection chemical feeding is to destroy pathogenic (disease-causing) organisms such as bacteria and viruses, with the purpose of rendering the receiving water safe for human use. Chlorine is typically used for this purpose. Because of chlorine's oxidizing nature, it is often used to condition other flows in a treatment plant. At Authority plants, chlorine can also be used for the control of odors in the influent sewage. Sulfur dioxide is needed to dechlorinate the final effluent before disposal.

The chlorine feed system consists of a liquid chlorine storage tank (normally a 1-ton cylinder from an outside supplier), two hot water bath evaporators, three vacuum type gas chlorinators, and associated nonpotable water facilities. Liquid chlorine is evaporated into a gas and fed as appropriate by the gas chlorinators into the flow entering the disinfection contact tank (see Figure 2.2). The sulfur dioxide feed system is identical to the chlorine feed system (see Figure 2.3).

Note: Sulfur dioxide feed equipment uses the same principles as chlorination equipment and requires the same components.

Note: In the summary of the theory of operation of chlorine feed system used at the Authority plants, the DST obtained the following information from the manufacturer's technical manual.

Evaporator: Liquid chlorine from the source containers is piped to the chlorine chamber. This chamber is immersed in a constant temperature hot water bath. The bath supplies the heat to convert the liquid to chlorine gas. Liquid enters the chamber through the top, but a drop pipe inside carries the liquid almost to the bottom. The alternate inlet connection at the bottom has a riser that terminates at approximately the same level as the drop pipe. The vapor outlet connection at the top also has a drop pipe, but it is not as long as the inlet drop pipe. Thus, the liquid chlorine enters near the bottom of the chamber, and the vapor leaves from a point somewhat below the top. This arrangement limits cylinder pressure to that of the source container and prevents the complete filling of the chamber with liquid chlorine. The heat transfer surface in the gas-filled portion of the cylinder superheats the chlorine vapor.

The liquid chlorine level in the cylinder is inherently self-adjusting to the chlorine gas removal rate. With a constant withdrawal rate, the liquid will assume a constant level. If the rate of gas withdrawal is increased, the gas pressure in the cylinder will be reduced. The liquid will then rise in the cylinder because of the supply pressure. This exposes more liquid to the transfer surface, where it will evaporate faster to meet the new demand. The gas pressure builds up until it equals the supply pressure, and the liquid level

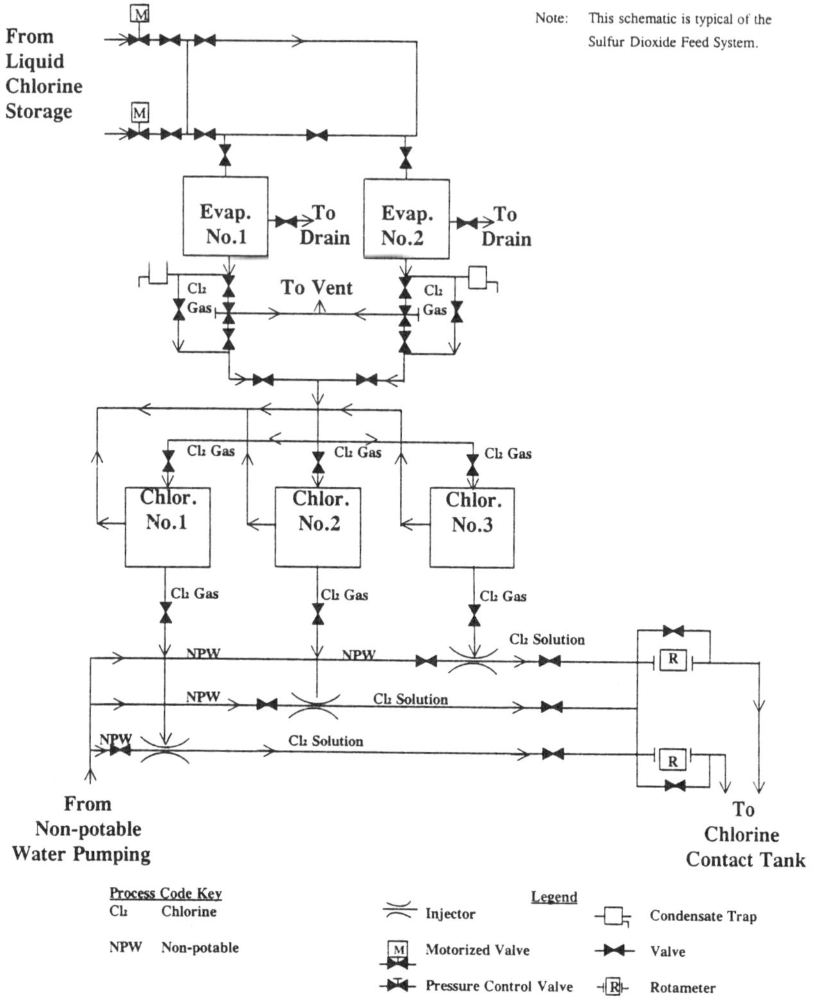

Figure 2.3 Disinfection chemical feeding process schematic diagram. (*Note:* This schematic is typical of the sulfur dioxide feed system.)

is restored to equilibrium. Similarly, a reduction in the withdrawal rate causes an increase in gas pressure, which lowers the liquid level, the amount of liquid exposed to the heat transfer surface, and consequently, the rate of evaporation.

Chlorinator/Sulfonator: The chlorinator operates under a vacuum produced by a flow of water through an aspirator type injector. The hydraulic conditions of the installation must ensure that the injector can produce a vacuum of at least 5 inches of mercury.

Chlorine/sulfur dioxide gas under pressure enters the chlorinator at the chlorine inlet connection, where it is electrically heated to reduce the deposit of impurities and to prevent reliquefication of the gas when the chlorinator is shut down with the chlorine supply turned on. A vacuum exerts pull on the diaphragm in the gas pressure regulating valve and opens the inlet valve. The entrance of chlorine will hold this vacuum at a fairly constant value. The vacuum on the upstream side of the V-notch variable orifice is somewhat higher because of the drop, through the rotameter, which depends on the rotameter capacity and the actual feed rate. The vacuum-regulating valve is designed to maintain a constant drop across the V-notch variable orifice. Thus, the flow through the orifice is entirely a function of the size of the orifice as determined by the position of the V-notch plug as manually set by the operator. From the vacuum-regulating valve, gas passes to the injector where it is mixed with water. The resultant solution is discharged to the point of application.

The pressure-vacuum relief valve serves a dual purpose. Should the chlorine supply be exhausted or shut off, or should the vacuum regulating valve fail to function properly, the vacuum on the upstream side of the V-notch orifice will increase. When a predetermined vacuum higher than the maximum normal operating vacuum develops, the diaphragm in the pressure-vacuum relief valve is pulled to open the valve stem and admit air from the vent to relieve the excess vacuum in the system. If the chlorine pressure-regulating valve does not seat properly and a slight positive pressure is developed in the chlorinator, the diaphragm in the pressure-vacuum relief valve is forced in the opposite direction, and the pressure is relieved through the diaphragm and then the vent. This is the reason why the vent line should be run to outside atmosphere.

After they looked over the unit process operation, the DST felt they had enough information on chlorine and the chlorine feed process used by the Authority. They needed to start summarizing the information they had gathered into something "usable"—something that they would be able to include in the final write-up that would eventually be presented to the GM.

The DST decided to put the USEPA's matrix for determining the applicability of alternative disinfection techniques to work (see Table 2.1). Using the EPA's format, they inserted information about elemental chlorine into the matrix (see Table 2.2).

The DST summarized their findings on the practicality of using elemental chlorine and sulfur dioxide for dechlorination at Rachel's Creek WWTP in a written preliminary report. (*Note:* The final report would not be possible until all the alternatives had been studied.) The chairperson felt the best format to use for this summary was to describe both the advantages and disadvantages of the elemental chlorine alternative as succinctly as possible in the DST's preliminary summary on elemental chlorine.

TABLE 2.2. Matrix for Determining the Applicability of Alternative Disinfection Techniques.

Alternative Disinfection Technique (e.g., Cl_2, BrCl, and O_3)	
Consideration	Elemental Chlorine
Size of plant	Suitable for all levels
Applicable level of treatment prior to disinfection	All levels
Equipment reliability	Fair to good
Process control	Well developed
Relative complexity of technology	Simple to moderate
Safety concerns—transportation on-site	Yes substantial
Bactericidal	Good
Virucidal	Poor
Fish toxicity	Toxic
Hazardous by-products	Yes
Persistent residual	Long
Contact time	Long
Contributes D.O.	No
Reacts with ammonia	Yes
Color removal	Moderate
Increased dissolved solids	Yes
pH dependent	Yes
O & M sensitive	Minimal
Corrosive	Yes
Covered by PSM/RMP	Yes (both chlorine and sulfur dioxide covered—Rachel's Creek would have to be in full compliance with the regulations)

2.2.7 SUMMARY STATEMENT: APPLICABILITY OF ELEMENTAL CHLORINE USE

- Elemental chlorine disinfection has been successfully used at the Authority for at least 35 years.
- Chlorine disinfection has several advantages: cost, dependability, and predictable performance.
- Chlorine and sulfur dioxide supplies are readily available locally.
- Although increased safety and regulatory requirements have increased operation and liability costs, chlorine remains relatively inexpensive compared with other disinfection methods.
- Chlorination equipment has been used for years, and as a result, designs are dependable. This reduces breakdowns and helps to ensure that when problems do occur, minimal time will be required to identify and correct the problem.

- The performance of the chlorine disinfection process is well documented and has an easy-to-use control mechanism (residual and contact time).
- The Authority's plant operators have several years' experience working with both chlorine and sulfur dioxide.
- The Authority has never (to date) had a chlorine incident [a release above the reportable quantity (RQ)]; several incidental leaks have occurred, all below the RQ.
- Chlorine/sulfur dioxide equipment replacement parts are readily available from local suppliers.
- Chlorine disinfection also has disadvantages: environmental impact and in-plant hazards.
- Chlorine produces chloramines and other substances, which, even when present in very low concentrations, are toxic to fish and aquatic organisms. Many of these compounds remain active in the receiving stream for very long periods. For this reason, many State Water Control Boards (including ours) established chlorine water quality standards of total residual chlorine ≤0.011 mg/L in fresh waters and ≤0.0075 mg/L for chlorine-produced oxidants in saline waters.
- Chlorine also produces by-products that are harmful to humans [trihalomethanes (THMs)] and that require additional treatment steps before the water can be reused.
- Because chlorine is an extremely toxic material, extra safety precautions, personal protective equipment, emergency response plans, considerable training time, and additional regulatory monitoring and reporting are required.

The major disadvantage of elemental chlorine and sulfur dioxide use (without a doubt) is the requirement to comply with USEPA's Risk Management Program (RMP). Although RMP is designed to ensure safer workplaces and to protect the public from the hazards of covered chemicals during a catastrophic release event, the additional requirements on the Authority (including all Authority facilities presently using elemental chlorine and sulfur dioxide) to be in full compliance with RMP are burdensome and costly. For all RMP compliance requirements listed here, see Section 1.4.2).

As far as the DST was concerned, the preliminary report on the applicability or nonapplicability of elemental chlorine as the disinfection unit process of choice was completed. After all the other alternatives had been studied, the DST would put together a final report, along with its recommendation.

The chairperson stated that when they reconvened the DST the following week, their focus of study would shift from elemental chlorine to the hypochlorite alternative. Then she dismissed the members of the DST.

After the DST members had departed from the conference room, Nancy Jo sat and reread the preliminary summary on elemental chlorine for the third time. "Something is missing," she told herself. "Something is missing . . . we have forgotten something." But what that something was escaped her.

Have you ever been assigned to do a task that you go ahead and complete, but when it is finished and you put it aside to move on to other "bigger and better" things, you have the heavy, nagging feeling that something isn't right? That you have forgotten something important? Have you been there? That's where Nancy Jo was now. In fact, she had been uncomfortable since the DST had completed its preliminary report on the chlorine alternative, 3 days earlier.

In her gut and subconscious she knew, felt, and realized that she and they had forgotten something important.

She continued her normal routine work activities for the rest of the week, knowing that the DST would reconvene on Monday and start working on the hypochlorite study. She knew this, but still that persistent, nagging feeling remained. She tried to brush it off several times but was as successful as one might be in removing an old tattoo with soap and water.

The missing piece popped into her mind Saturday night. She now knew what she and they forgot. Later, she couldn't believe she had forgotten such a critical piece of the puzzle. What was the missing piece? A nationwide survey, of course.

To add credibility to the DST's findings in its final report, the ultimate presentation to the GM, she needed hard, cold, precise facts. What better facts could one gather than real-world evidence of what the "other guys" (other WWTP's) nationwide were doing? She realized that anybody and everybody presently using elemental chlorine at levels above RMP threshold quantity value (≥2,500) lb, for whatever purpose, were facing the same dilemma as the Authority: to stay with elemental chlorine and comply fully with RMP or to substitute some chemical or process that is not RMP-covered.

How should she implement the survey? She devised her plan with the following points:

- As member (and so is the Authority) of one of the world's largest professional wastewater treatment associations, The World Wastewater Federation (WWF), I know that just about every WWTP (POTW), Sanitation Authority, Sanitation District, etc. in the United States has membership as well. I have their addresses and a key point of contact (POC): a real person.
- I need to come up with a list (actually narrow down the list from 16,000 POTWs) of 250 POTWs nationwide, which should give me a representative sample.

- I need to develop a survey form that asks the right questions in a relatively simple form and style (see below).

Her survey form was actually almost a memo more than anything else. Take a look at what the DST chairperson developed:

Dear WWF Member,

The Sanitation Authority of Rachel's Creek is in the process of randomly surveying 250 POTWs nationwide to make a determination of how these facilities intend to comply with USEPA's Risk Management Program (RMP), regarding the chemicals and processes used for water/wastewater disinfection. Some of you might not be covered under RMP, for whatever reason.

I have made this survey form as simple as possible. Please answer the following questions and mail your response back to me in the self-addressed, stamped envelope as soon as you can.

When the results of the survey are analyzed and tabulated, I will send each respondent a copy of the findings.

Please circle and/or fill-in the correct response:

(1) Do you plan to stay with elemental chlorine and/or sulfur dioxide? Yes or No

(2) Do you plan to substitute chlorine with a noncovered chemical or process? Yes or No
If so, which chemical or process are you substituting? ____________

(3) Have you decided to do anything yet? Yes or No

Thank you for your participation.

Chairperson
Disinfection Selection Team
Sanitation Authority
Rachel's Creek WWTP

On Monday, before beginning their discussion and research on the hypochlorite alternative, Nancy Jo gave each member a copy of her survey letter and waited for their comments. The DST members agreed with the chairperson that the survey was a good idea, and they made no changes to her format. Later that day, the chairperson had her assistant mail all 250 surveys.

That evening, the chairperson thought about the surveys. She realized that not all 250 POTWs would respond to the survey. However, she was hoping that at least 50% would. She also realized that weeks could go by before she had all the responses that she was going to get, but that did not bother her, because she still had seven disinfection alternatives to examine and 43 days to complete the entire study. Even with so little time left, she knew the team had enough time. The alternatives left to be studied would not take as long as the elemental chlorine study did; at least, this is how she viewed the situation at present.

In the end, she was proven correct.

2.3 REFERENCES

Chicago Daily Herald (Timothy S. Rooney), July 1998.

Lehrer, T. *That Was the Year That Was.* Reprise Records R6179, 1965.

The Commercial Appeal (Tom Charlier), Memphis, TN, April 1998.

USEPA. *Design Manual: Municipal Wastewater Disinfection*, 1986.

White, G. C. *Handbook of Chlorination* (2nd ed.). New York: Van Nostrand Reinhold, 1986.

CHAPTER 3

Hypochlorite

. . . See the halibuts and the sturgeons
Being wiped out by detergeons. (Tom Lehrer, 1965)

3.1 SETTING THE STAGE

On Monday morning, the DST was back in session. On Friday afternoon, the chairperson had requested the Authority's Safety Director (the DST's recorder) to prepare a short introduction—a "biographical sketch" for hypochlorite. Nancy Jo also requested that such an introduction be provided for all the subsequent disinfection alternatives to be discussed.

The Safety Director presented the following "biographical sketch" on hypochlorite.

- Hypochlorite (see Figure 3.1) is about three times the strength of common household bleach—strong, but not highly hazardous like chlorine.
- Although some hazards are associated with hypochlorite use (skin irritation, nose irritation, and burning eyes), it is relatively safe to work with. Normally available in dry form, as pellet or tablet calcium hypochlorite, or in liquid sodium hypochlorite form, it can be added directly by using a dry chemical feeder or dissolved and fed as a solution.
- Hypochlorites are salts of hypochlorous acid. Several grades are available, but sodium hypochlorite ($NaOCl$) is the only liquid hypochlorite form in current use. Calcium hypochlorite [$Ca(OCl)_2$] is the predominant dry form.
- Sodium hypochlorite is often referred to as liquid bleach or Javelle water. Available in liquid form only, it typically is sold in concentrations between 5 and 15% available chlorine. Tinted yellow, solutions are strongly alkaline and corrosive, with a strong chlorinous odor.

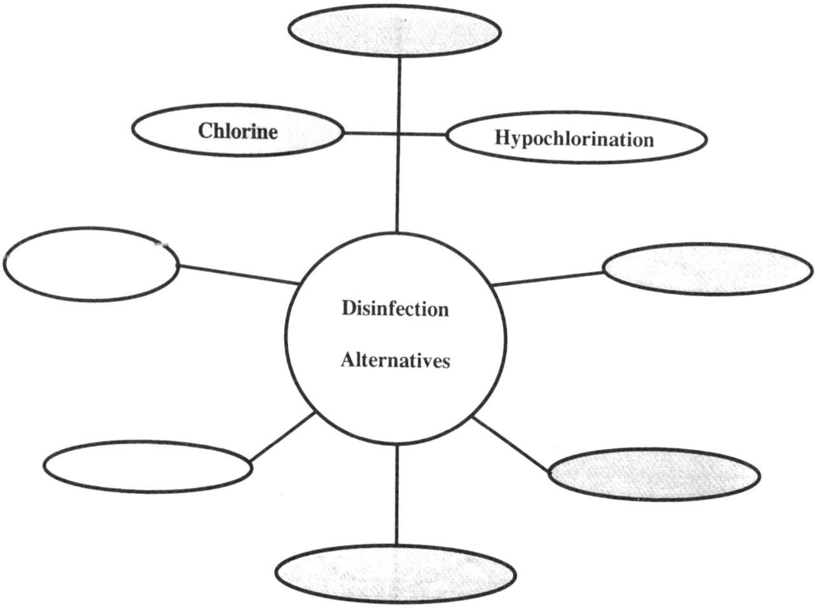

Figure 3.1 Hypochlorination alternative.

- Calcium hypochlorite is a white, hygroscopic, dry material, commonly referred to as powder bleach or high-test hypochlorite (HTH). It typically consists of 65% available chlorine. $Ca(OCl)_2$ emits a strong, chlorinous odor.
- Hypochlorites are very strong oxidants. Sodium hypochlorite solutions are unstable. Heat, light, storage time, and impurities such as iron accelerate product degradation. Calcium hypochlorite is unstable under normal atmospheric conditions. When mixed with turpentine, oils, water, or paper, reactions may occur spontaneously; thus, calcium hypochlorite must be stored in dry locations and used only with equipment free of organics.

The use of hypochlorite would allow Rachel's Creek to avoid RMP-related expenses and compliance requirements, although it is about two to three times as costly as the equivalent strength of chlorine in ton cylinders.

3.2 THE PLUSES/MINUSES OF HYPOCHLORITE

On completing his brief introductory presentation on hypochlorite, the Safety Director displayed a new set of flip charts (a clean slate) and prepared to list the items he and the team provided on the information they gathered from their own "local" knowledge and from their research on hypochlorite.

3.2.1 BASIC INFORMATION

- sodium hypochlorite
  —symbol, NaOCl
  —form, liquid
  —strength, up to 15% available chlorine
  —clear, greenish-yellow liquid
  —stored in cool, dry, dark location in tightly sealed container
- calcium hypochlorite
  —symbol, $Ca(OCl)_2$
  —form, dry granules, powder, or tablets
  —strength, 65–70% available chlorine, depending on form
  —10 lb contains 6.5 lb available chlorine
  —can burn if mixed with oil, grease, etc.
  —stored cool and dry in air tight container

3.2.2 SODIUM HYPOCHLORITE VERSUS CALCIUM HYPOCHLORITE

At this point in the proceedings, the Safety Director paused to change directions. Jake proposed that they consider only sodium hypochlorite disinfection as a viable alternative within the varieties of hypochlorites. He explained that local suppliers of sodium hypochlorite were available, whereas calcium hypochlorite would have to be shipped in from some distance, increasing overall costs. In addition, the Safety Director explained that one significant disadvantage in using calcium hypochlorite is that it requires manual handling of the tablets, as well as other handling problems. He pointed out that although sodium hypochlorite requires more storage space than calcium hypochlorite does, sodium hypochlorite handles more easily and creates fewer maintenance problems with pumping and metering equipment. "Besides," he stated, "liquid sodium hypochlorite systems have been in use for many years and have an established operational history—a track record."

The DST considered the Safety Director's suggestion and voted to approve it; their focus was to be on sodium hypochlorite.

3.2.3 SODIUM HYPOCHLORITE: GENERAL INFORMATION

- Liquid sodium hypochlorite reduces the risk of a chlorine leak because it is a liquid. It typically does not produce toxic vapors when spilled.
- Liquid sodium hypochlorite is available in 15-gallon carboys,

55-gallon drums, intermediate bulk tanks of 300 to 500 gallons, and bulk quantities.

- Sodium hypochlorite systems have been used for many years and are covered under current design standards for water and wastewater treatment plants.
- The choice of the sodium hypochlorite alternative over elemental chlorine would add an undetermined amount to Authority's treatment costs, because sodium hypochlorite is more expensive. But, again, the hypochlorite, which simply carries chlorine in a liquid, is equally as effective in killing bacteria and microbes and is safer to handle than the gas. In addition, hypochlorite reduces the Authority's worry about the public relations fallout from the worst-case scenario maps required for chlorine.
- Not only is sodium hypochlorite not on the EPA list, it is also safer to handle.
- Sodium hypochlorite is manufactured by the reaction of molecular chlorine with sodium hydroxide and water. A small excess of sodium hydroxide is required to maintain the pH between 11 and 13 to minimize decomposition.
- Sodium hypochlorite has long been recognized as having outstanding disinfection properties. It has been proven by the Institute Pasteur in Paris to be the most effective disinfectant against all known pathogenic bacteria, fungi and viruses (Fletcher and Ciancone, 1996).
- Installing or converting to sodium hypochlorite alleviates most of the safety concerns associated with storing and using gaseous chlorine. However, it does not address the negative impact of chlorinated compounds on water and air quality. Because of its nonselectivity, NaOCl reacts rapidly with organics as well as H_2S. This is an important point, because most odor control chemical addition is done to raw sewage (collection system or plant headworks) where the organic load is relatively high. The aforementioned side reactions result in increased hypochlorite usage and the formation of chlorinated by-products, which may be toxic or refractory to biological treatment.
- Sodium hypochlorite is very corrosive and should be stored with care and kept away from equipment that can be damaged by corrosion. Hypochlorite solutions decompose rapidly and should not be stored for more than 1 month. They must be stored in a cool, dark, dry area.
- Because the Authority is required to dechlorinate its wastewater effluent, sodium bisulfite will be required in place of the sulfur dioxide used to dechlorinate elemental chlorine.
- Hypochlorite concentration conventions
  —trade % (as Cl_2): mg/L/10,000; example: 150,000 mg/L = "15% hypochlorite"

—actual concentration (weight basis): trade %/S.G.; example: 15% trade/1.25 = 12% Cl_2

- Equivalent chlorine
  —NaOCl (sodium ions and hypochlorite ions in solutions)
  —expressed as equivalent chlorine; 15% (trade = 1.25 lb Cl_2/gal; 12.5% (trade) = 1.0 lb Cl_2/gal
- Hypochlorite decomposition
  —$2OCl^- + 2Na^+ \Rightarrow O_2 + 2Na^+ + 2Cl^-$
- Factors affecting the degradation of sodium hypochlorite
  —metals (iron, cobalt, mercury, copper)
  —heat
  —UV light
- Effects of decomposition
  —loss of chemical strength
  —accelerated corrosion (more aggressive environment)
  —offgassing
- Solution stability
  —second-order reaction (rate of decomposition proportional to square of concentration): $dC/dt = -kC^2$
- Design considerations
  —protect tanks from sunlight and heat
  —vent pump suctions and discharges
  —suction strainers
  —pulsation dampeners
  —maximize suction head
  —tank venting
- Materials of construction
  —acceptable materials: titanium, Hastelloy C, FRP, PVC/CPVC, Teflon, EPDM, and Hypalon
  —poor or unacceptable materials: 316 SST, GRPP, Kynar (PVDF), Viton
- In use, hypochlorite solution must not be contaminated with bits of metal and other contaminants. They can jam pump check valves and plug strainers. The hypochlorite solution must be inspected to ensure that it is yellow and clear.

3.3 SODIUM HYPOCHLORITE SYSTEM

Sodium hypochlorite systems typically consist of storage tanks, metering pumps, and a control system to adjust chlorine dosage in response to plant flow and chlorine residual (see Figure 3.2). Enough storage should be provided for 30 days at average design demand. Because of decomposition, storing the smallest volume possible (as long as hypochlorite delivery is

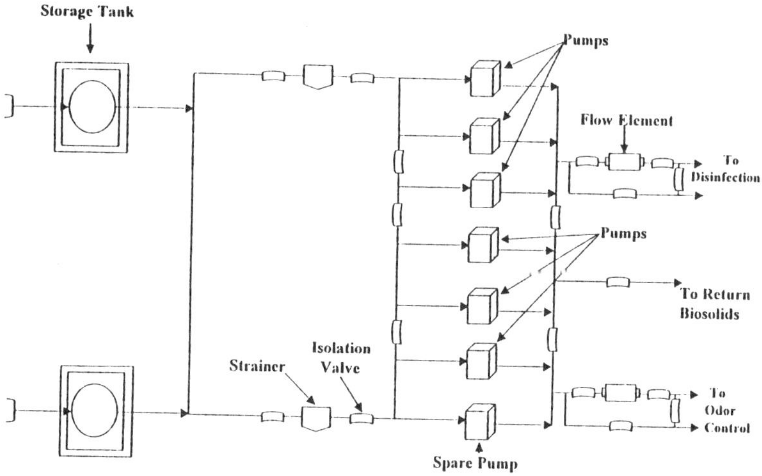

Figure 3.2 Process flow diagram sodium hypochlorite.

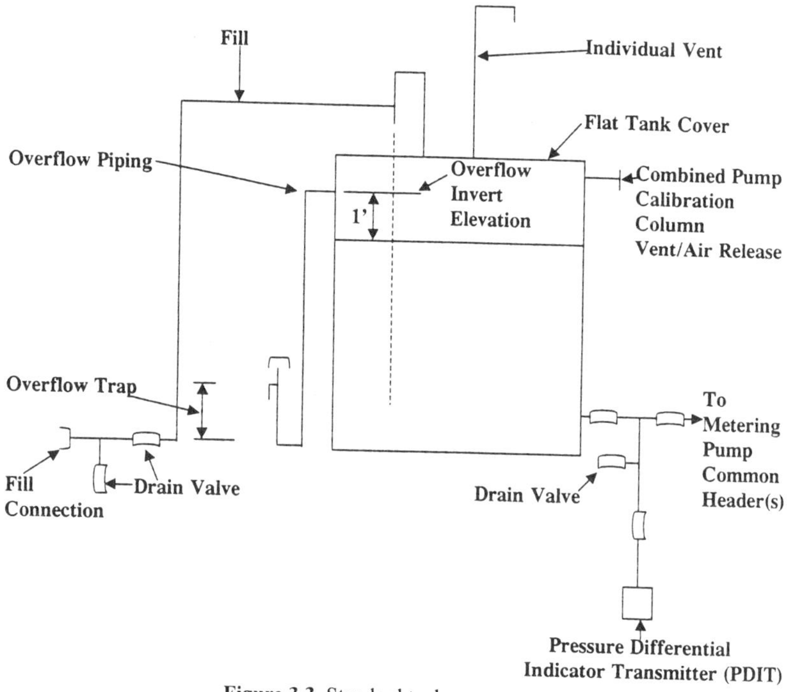

Figure 3.3 Standard tank arrangement.

reliable) is the most effective practice. Extra tanks should be installed to ensure chemical feed is maintained while filling or servicing off-line units. The volume of an individual tank should be at least 25% greater than anticipated tank delivery volume, so that the entire delivery can be received. When calculating this volume, we must account for solution decomposition.

The best tanks presently available for storing sodium hypochlorite are filament-wound FRP tanks (fiberglass reinforced plastic; see Figure 3.3). Tanks should also have a laminate configuration—an inner surface layer, an inner corrosion barrier, and an external layer with a pigmented gel coat containing UV inhibitors. Maximum tank diameter is about 12 feet (Voutchkov, 1995).

The best type of chemical metering pumps for use with sodium hypochlorite are positive displacement, hydraulically actuated with double diaphragms (see Figure 3.4).

PVC piping has proven successful for conveying sodium hypochlorite (as long as it is kept within temperature and pressure limitations).

Sodium hypochlorite and sodium bisulfite systems use the same control strategies as those used by chlorine and sulfur dioxide systems. Control systems can employ traditional feed forward, feedback, or compound loop strategies (Walkowiak et al., 1996).

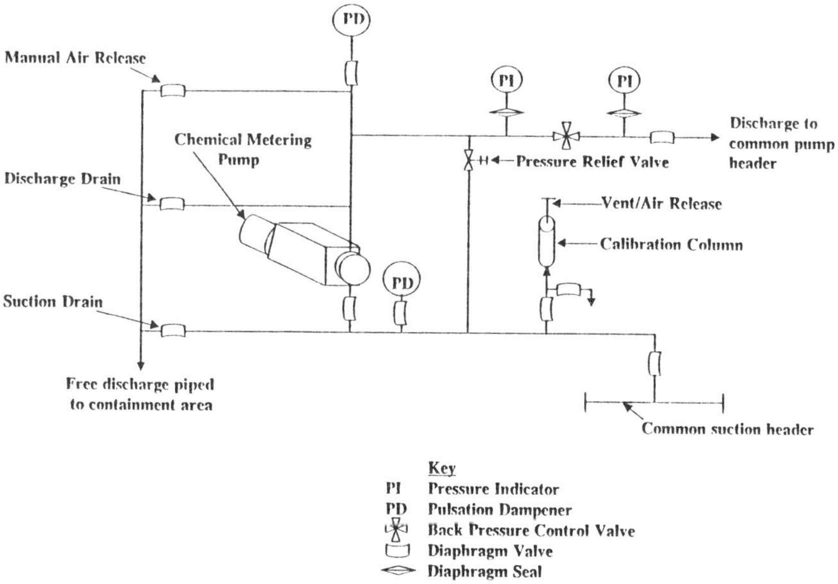

Figure 3.4 Standard chemcial metering pump arrangement.

3.4 SODIUM HYPOCHLORITE: SAFETY CONSIDERATIONS

- Sodium hypochlorite is safer to handle than gaseous chlorine.
- Sodium hypochlorite is inherently unstable and loses about one-half of its strength every 100 days at 21°C.
- Sodium hypochlorite degradation occurring from contamination, light, or heat can produce oxygen gas and sodium chlorate. Oxygen and/or sodium chlorate formation can lead to a fire or explosion hazard from the oxygen release or the sodium chlorate, if the sodium chlorate is allowed to dry or comes in contact with acids and organic materials.
- Hazardous conditions can also develop from a sudden decrease in pH caused by accidentally mixing sodium hypochlorite solution with ferric chloride, ammonia, or other acidic compounds. Precautions should be taken to prevent possible mixing of these or other incompatible materials.
- Because of the catalytic reactions caused by metal contamination and chlorine off-gassing that occurs as the solution's pH decreases, hypochlorite purchase specifications should be written to require a maximum metals content of 0.5 mg/L iron and 1.0 mg/L copper and a pH range between 11.0 and 11.2 (White, 1992).
- Sodium hydroxide and sodium bisulfite storage tanks (see Figure 3.5) must be isolated and diked off or contained within cement containment structures. In addition, pumps and piping between tanks also must be contained, so that failure of an individual pipe or wall penetration cannot cause the entire tank contents to spill. The exact containment volume must be factored in by the design engineers; the minimum volume, however, should be enough to contain the contents of the largest tank in the event of a major spill.
- Even though sodium hypochlorite is less dangerous than chlorine gas, it is a corrosive chemical and must be handled carefully.
- PPE requirements include gloves, eye protection, and aprons during handling.
- Deluge showers and eyewashes should be strategically placed within easy reach near storage and metering pump areas.
- One of the greatest hazards associated with sodium hypochlorite is the possibility that it will come into contact with incompatibles such as acids, which cause chlorine gas to be liberated. In addition, sodium hypochlorite reacts violently with organic compounds such as greases, oils, and fuels.
- It is absolutely essential that only hypochlorite can be put into a hypochlorite storage tank. G. C. White (1992) emphatically makes this point in his account of an incident that occurred in Knoxville, Tennessee, in April 1983. In this instance, a truck driver delivering

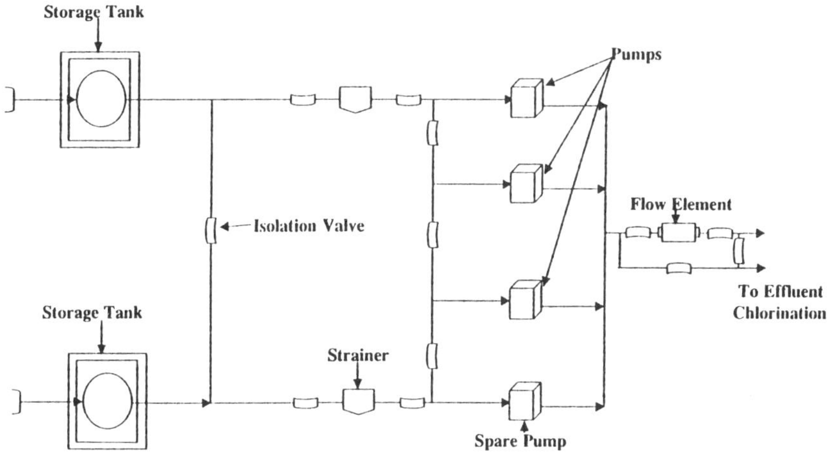

Figure 3.5 Process flow diagram sodium bisulfate.

ferric chloride to a plant he was not familiar with inadvertently connected the delivery hose to the sodium hypochlorite tank. He pumped about 600 gallons of ferric chloride into the tank, which contained about 3,000 gallons of sodium hypochlorite. Immediately, the two substances reacted, and molecular chlorine was produced and released from the hypochlorite. Chlorine gas rolled out of the hypochlorite vent in a lethal cloud. Fortunately, local HazMat responders handled the incident correctly, and proper evacuation of the area was effected with no loss of life. This incident could not have occurred if the connections to the two tanks (ferric chloride and sodium hypochlorite) had been different.

3.5 SODIUM HYPOCHLORITE: OTHER CONSIDERATIONS

By the close of business on Tuesday, most of the DST members felt they had enough information on sodium hypochlorite to enable them to insert data into their standard matrix and to write up a summary of their findings. However, Nancy Jo did not share this view. As chairperson, she felt that sodium hypochlorite might end up being their disinfection alternative of choice; the fact that they would not have to comply with RMP and the Authority's concern over public relations were strong selling points, but she was uncomfortable with the extent of the information they had gathered to this point.

During the research and discussion phase for sodium hypochlorite, she had come up with an idea. A friend of hers was the plant manager for a

POTW called Nancy's Run in the upper northeastern part of the state. Nancy Jo knew that Nancy's Run had been using hypochlorite and bisulfite for several years to disinfect and dechlorinate the treated effluent from the plant. On Tuesday morning, she called and asked permission to send the prospective plant manager and superintendent to Nancy's Run to get the 411 on sodium hypochlorite use at Nancy's Run. Nancy's Run Plant Manager granted permission, so Nancy Jo directed Rachel's Creek prospective plant manager and superintendent to drive up to the plant site on Wednesday and to spend all day Thursday gathering operational facts. The two Rachel's Creek employees were to report back both in writing and orally to the DST. The DST recorder would make their written report part of the DST's report on disinfection alternatives.

While the two Rachel's Creek employees were up north, the chairperson directed the rest of the DST members to start gathering data on chloramines, the disinfection alternative they would research and discuss the next week. In the meantime, Nancy Jo had some studying to do on her own.

On Friday morning, the DST reconvened. The prospective plant manager of Rachel's Creek handed each member of the DST a copy of his written findings at Nancy's Run. These findings became part of the DST's overall report, and are included in their entirety here.

3.5.1 SODIUM HYPOCHLORITE USE AT NANCY'S RUN POTW

Nancy's Run Wastewater Treatment Plant converted from using gaseous chlorine for disinfection to using sodium hypochlorite 4 years ago. Nancy's Run made the conversion to hypochlorite (as many plants across the country have also been designed or retrofitted to use hypochlorite) for various reasons, mostly to provide a way of escaping the heavy hand the regulators used to enforce RMP. Plant management at Nancy's Run was also worried about the public perception of the hazards associated with gaseous chlorine at the plant site. The assumption was that hypochlorite is just chlorine already dissolved in water and that past design practices used with chlorine gas could also be applied to hypochlorite. Nancy's Run found that this was not the case. In this report, we outline the problems they found and some of the solutions they have developed at Nancy's Run.

Nancy's Run WWTP, a 60 MGD secondary treatment facility, was converted from gaseous chlorine to hypochlorite by two different engineering firms, primarily to eliminate the risks associated with storage and usage of chlorine gas.

The system in the original chlorine gas installation was typical of most. Chlorine gas was dissolved into water at low concentrations as needed by the process. The dilute solution of chlorine in water was delivered to the point of application. The controls used adjusted the amount of gas introduced into the carry water. To minimize costs, retrofits at Nancy's Run used the same delivery system, substituting hypochlorite pumps for the vacuum injectors. Sodium hypochlorite is manufactured by injecting chlorine gas into a solution of caustic (sodium hydroxide) at a high pH. At a high pH, chlorine gas is much more soluble and can be made into a percent (% by volume) solution.

After 1 year of operation, Nancy's Run encountered several problems with the hypochlorite installation. As time passed and as they gained experience, these problems were resolved, but only after many "lessons-learned." We provide these "lessons-learned" in this report. Specifically, the plant's major problems stemmed from around six separate problems: leakage, scaling, gas production, mixing, storage, and safety and corrosion.

3.5.1.1 Nancy's Run: Leakage Problem

Nancy's Run first encountered leakage of neat (undiluted) hypochlorite when glued PVC and threaded fittings began to leak frequently. From experience, they discovered that a tiny water leak normally evaporates, leaving no sign of leakage. However, hypochlorite is so aggressive because of its high pH and chlorine content that it exploits any and every weak spot. Because it is so concentrated, a pile of salts builds up at every tiny leak (its caustic content pulls carbon dioxide from the air to make an even bigger pile of sodium carbonate). One of the problems Nancy's Run discovered was caused by the work practices of the pipefitters. Most of them installed PVC fittings by slapping some primer on, then glue, then shoving the fittings together. Sometimes this practice worked, but usually it did not. To avoid this problem, pipefitters had to be trained to properly fit PVC piping and connectors, following the manufacturer's guidelines to the letter.

For threaded joints, Nancy's Run discovered (through trial and error) that not all grades of Teflon tape are the same. They recommend avoiding the cheaper grades sold at hardware stores and using only Mil spec P-27730A rated grade.

3.5.1.2 Scaling

To maintain the chlorine in solution, sodium hydroxide (caustic) is used to raise the pH of the hypochlorite; the excess caustic raises the shelf life. A high pH caustic solution raises the pH of the dilution water to over pH 9.0 after dilution. The calcium in the dilution water reacts with dissolved CO_2 and forms calcium carbonate. Two-inch pipes at Nancy's Run turned into 3/4-inch pipes from scale buildup. The scale deposition is greatest in areas of turbulence such as pumps, valves, rotameters and backpressure devices.

If lime (calcium oxide) is added for alkalinity, plant water used as dilution water will have higher calcium levels and generate more scale. At present, Nancy's Run has approximately 48 mg/L of calcium in their effluent. Their diluted hypochlorite (1:50) generates 82 mg of scale per liter in lab experiments. Although softened water will not generate scale, it is also true that it is expensive in large quantities. Nancy's Run uses softened water on hypochlorite mist odor scrubbers only.

Scaling also occurred in solution rotameters, making flow readings impossible and freezing the flow indicator in place. In addition, various valves froze up, and pressure-sustaining valves froze and plugged. Various small diffuser holes also filled with scale. To slow the rate of scaling, Nancy's Run purchases water from a local township at a cost of about $27,500 per year to dilute hypochlorite for the RAS and miscellaneous uses.

Nancy's Run also experimented by not adding lime to the system. When they did this, manganese dioxide (black deposits) developed on the rotameters glass, making viewing the float impossible. Then they moved the point of hypochlorite addition to downstream of the rotameter, which seemed to solve the problem.

They also had three large (3-inch) 1,400-foot-long delivery lines scale up. (*Note:* Detention time in the lines was significant at 30 hours.) To avoid additional scaling, Nancy's Run delivered only neat (undiluted) hypochlorite in them. To date, this seems to have been a positive decision.

3.5.1.3 Gas Production

Over time, hypochlorite loses strength and degrades, generating gas. Nancy's Run estimates that at normal room temperature, their system was producing about 1% gas per day. One pound of gas per day was produced from every 100 gallons of hypochlorite. Surprisingly (to nonchemists, anyway), the gas produced is not chlorine, but instead, oxygen. Chlorine gas is only produced when the pH is low. What happens is that the ^{-}OCl ions collide and generate oxygen gas and two chloride ions. The chloride ion has no ability to disinfect.

$$H^{+}\ ^{-}OCl + H^{+}\ ^{-}OCl \rightarrow O_2 + 2HCl$$

The reaction rate increases with concentration, temperature, and catalysts. Because of this, hypochlorite should be stored in a cool location, for as short a time as possible, with no metal contact. In any case, exposure to the sun is not a good idea.

In the 1,400 ft, 3-inch delivery lines mentioned earlier, gas from decomposition accumulated in high spots and made delivery somewhat erratic. Nancy's Run calculated that 0.7 cubic feet of gas was generated each day in the pipe, by the pipe contents. They replaced the large delivery lines with 3/8-inch lines delivering neat hypochlorite. The smaller lines work to move the hypochlorite faster, so gas bubbles are literally swept downstream. The smaller sized piping also reduces detention time (1.6-hour detention time as opposed to the previous 30 hours). They also found that excess glue had plugged some 3/8-inch lines initially because the glue brush used was too large for the application. They switched to a smaller size brush for small pipes. Reducing stress on the pipes by securing them to larger pipes or laying them in a gallery tray is also important.

The most critical problem with gas produced from hypochlorite degradation, along with its production in the first place, is when it occurs in a restricted space, where the gas builds up pressure. In one incident at Nancy's Run, a 4-inch schedule 80 PVC valve closed, trapping the hypochlorite in the hollow part of the ball. With nowhere to expand, the pressure built up and exploded the valve. In another instance, two large interconnected tanks had large ball valves in the line. In one situation, a valve was opened and then closed and left for too long a period of time. The gas buildup caused the trapped hypochlorite to explode, and both tanks drained. If we choose this option, we must ensure that we avoid ball valves that have not been vented to the downstream pipe. Instead, we should use diaphragm valves; they do not trap hypochlorite internally.

Another serious problem with hypochlorite pumps involves diaphragms that rupture for no apparent reason. During the repair process, they noticed that one of the pumps was registering 185 psi. With further investigation, they found that the pump discharge was valved off, and the pump check valves prevented the hypochlorite from discharging back to the tank. The hypochlorite was generating sufficient pressure to rupture the diaphragm. Even isolated pipe runs exploded on occasion. Either the hypochlorite lines need to be flushed before isolating, or long term isolation of hypochlorite lines should be avoided.

At one of the odor control stations, the hypochlorite pumps occasionally lost prime. The tank was located below grade in a pit, and the pumps had a suction lift. The suction worked to pull the dissolved gas out of solution and air locked the pumps. They solved this problem by installing a recirculation pump at the bottom of the tank to pump hypochlorite past the feed pumps and back into the tank. There is some history at other plants with large, level, suction lines that accumulated gas and air locked the pumps, even with a pressure head. Under these circumstances, they had the manufacturer reduce the headspace in the pumps so it would handle the accumulated gas. If we choose this option, we must ensure that we use the smallest line the flow rate will permit or vent back to the source tank if needed.

To prevent loss of hypochlorite from being an issue at Rachel's Creek, we should have the manufacturer deliver hypochlorite at strengths greater than the minimum specifications and keep our storage at between 10 and 15 days. The tanks should be built inside a building.

Note that hypochlorite strength is reduced by the formation of chlorates.

$$3NaOCl \rightarrow NaClO_3 + 2NaCl$$

Chlorates have no ability to disinfect and there are concerns about chlorate in drinking water.

3.5.1.4 Mixing

Nancy's Run found that using a diffusion header to mix hypochlorite at the point of application requires the addition of dilution water. This causes scale to build up in the diffuser and its orifices. They just replaced the unit, until they tried acid washing to deal with the scale. They found the best way to combat this problem is to use flash mixing to introduce neat hypochlorite into the flow stream. They also found that if the hypochlorite is diluted, scale builds up inside the mixer. The flash mixers they used applied a suction to pull gases or solution into the mixer. The suction caused gas to come out of solution in the neat hypochlorite and separate the column of hypochlorite into alternating segments of gas and hypochlorite in the line. This resulted in huge doses of hypochlorite being delivered, followed by a period of no hypochlorite delivery, until the pipe refilled with hypochlorite and the cycle repeated. They found that providing an air gap between the end of the hypochlorite delivery pipe and the flash mixer intake prevented erratic delivery.

3.5.1.5 Storage

Nancy's Run found that hypochlorite is hard on storage tanks; in fact, it's downright abusive. Although their tanks are not old enough to have experienced any serious problems, they have had a few less serious problems (e.g., minor leaks). Industrywide, we hear reports of fiberglass-reinforced plastic (FRP) tanks 6 to 9 years old that leak. Because of these industry problems, Nancy's Run modified their FRP tanks to include a 20 mil Nexus veil coating to increase life and to protect the fiberglass strands from contacting the hypochlorite and wicking it into the tank wall. With the Nexus lining, they have an estimated life of 7 to 10 years, depending on temperature and other variables. Nancy's Run inspects their tanks annually and has designed hatches in the roof of each tank to allow for replacement. Experience shows that these tanks usually fail at manway and segment joints. To repair the tanks, cracks are stress-relieved by drilling, and then a new veil coating is applied.

3.5.1.6 Safety and Corrosion

Hypochlorite lines under pressure and at strengths of 15% are a significant safety issue for operators. Personal protective equipment (PPE) such as safety goggles, gloves, and aprons are a must.

Corrosion also causes problems. When small leaks occur, liquid hypochlorite releases chlorine gas into the air, causing the surrounding materials to suffer from corrosion. Nancy's Run has had pumpheads fall off because the bolts holding them into place were not as corrosion-resistant as the pumphead material; these bolts were replaced with corrosion-resistant bolts.

Overall, even with the initial "bugs," Nancy's Run is pleased with the operation of their sodium hypochlorite system.

3.6 SODIUM HYPOCHLORITE: MATRIX

On Friday morning of that week, the DST felt that it had all the information it needed to complete its applicability matrix (see Table 3.1) and to put together a preliminary summary report on sodium hypochlorite. From the sodium hypochlorite matrix below, note that the only differences between the matrix for chlorine and sodium hypochlorite are the alternative considered and the last entry: covered by PSM/RMP. Sodium hypochlorite is not covered under RMP. The rest of the entries are the same, of course, because hypochlorite is a chlorination process.

3.6.1 SUMMARY STATEMENT: APPLICABILITY OF SODIUM HYPOCHLORITE USE

- Sodium hypochlorite for disinfection of wastewater effluent has been successfully used for many years. Sodium hypochlorite and sodium bisulfite systems are viable alternatives to chlorine and sulfur dioxide, but like any other disinfection system, must be carefully designed and operated properly.
- Sodium hypochlorite use will afford Rachel's Creek WWTP a way out from under compliance with RMP requirements, but it's not a perfect solution.
- Using sodium hypochlorite allows Rachel's Creek to avoid safety-related expenses, even though it is about two to three times as costly as the equivalent strength of chlorine in ton cylinders.
- Particular attention must be given to selecting construction materials and making system configuration decisions, because of the chemical properties of sodium hypochlorite and sodium bisulfite.
- To ensure proper design, construction, and operation, we need to

TABLE 3.1. Matrix for Determining the Applicability of Alternative Disinfection Techniques.

Alternative Disinfection Technique (e.g., Cl_2, BrCl, and O_3)	
Consideration	Sodium Hypochlorite
Size of plant	50 MGD (suitable for all levels)
Applicable level of treatment prior to disinfection	All levels
Equipment reliability	Fair to good
Process control	Well developed
Relative complexity of technology	Simple to moderate
Safety concerns—transportation on-site	Yes, substantial
Bactericidal	Good
Virucidal	Poor
Fish toxicity	Toxic
Hazardous by-products	Yes
Persistent residual	Long
Contact time	Long
Contributes D.O.	No
Reacts with ammonia	Yes
Color removal	Moderate
Increased dissolved solids	Yes
pH dependent	Yes
O & M sensitive	Minimal
Corrosive	Yes
Covered by PSM/RMP	No

apply the lessons learned by our counterparts (those who have been using sodium hypochlorite and sodium bisulfite for years).

- Sodium hypochlorite should be kept neat if possible; otherwise, the plant will have to replace lines as they scale up.
- Keep sodium hypochlorite lines as small as the flow rate will allow.
- Avoid unvented ball valves and provide a means to flush lines and equipment when they are taken out of service.
- Flash-mixing is recommended.
- The key to success in using sodium hypochlorite for disinfection is to keep the entire system as simple as possible.

That Friday evening, the belt of the treadmill rolled along steadily as Nancy Jo thought about the progress the DST had made this week. Along with chlorine the week before and hypochlorite this week, she felt the DST was right on schedule; next week chloramines . . . no problem, she told herself.

She also felt a sense of accomplishment. She felt the hardest part of the study was already behind them. Chlorine had to be dissected right down to the marrow, and it was. With the exception of actual costs, present worth, future worth, and other financial aspects, every other possible aspect related to substituting hypochlorite for chlorine had been considered. The others were still to be studied, but realistically, Nancy Jo was sure that in the end the ultimate decision would evolve around two alternatives: chlorine or hypochlorite.

As she finished her hour-long run, the contentment, peace, and satisfaction of a good workout on the treadmill washed over her. Finished, she sat on the stool and toweled off, her face wearing a broad smile. She was smiling because she felt good, because she knew her team was doing a top-notch job, because they were progressing along right on schedule, but also because the survey forms she had mailed out last Friday were starting to flow back to her. To date, out of the original 250 mailed, 23 had been returned. When she had reviewed them 2 hours earlier, she was not surprised to find that at least the early respondents had already accomplished their compliance effort by one means or another or were heading there, and most had completed the effort or were in the process of completing it. Her smile was generated, not from the early numbers of respondents, but from the fact that most of them had been or were thinking about the disinfection choices in the same manner in which she was; of those who had already determined their decision, most chose the alternative method that she was leaning toward choosing.

3.7 REFERENCES

Fletcher, J. and Ciancone, D. Why Life's a Bleach (The Sodium Hypochlorite Story), *ES&E*, May 1996.

Lehrer, T. *That Was the Year That Was,* Reprise Records R6179, 1965.

Voutchkov, N. Everything You Always Wanted to Know About Sodium Hypochlorite . . . but Were Afraid to Ask. *Operations Forum*, 12, 10, 20–24, 1995.

Walkowiak, M., et al. Real World Experience Using Sodium Hypochlorite/Bisulfite Disinfection Systems. Paper presented at *Water Environment Federation 69th Annual Conference and Exposition,* Dallas, Texas, 123–135, 1996.

White, G. C. *Handbook of Chlorination* (2nd ed.). New York: Van Nostrand Reinhold, 1992.

3.8 SUGGESTED READING

American Water Works Association. *AWWA Standard for Hypochlorite.* ANSI/AWWA B300–92, 1992.

Baur, R. *Hypochlorite Problems and Some Solutions.* Tigard, OR: Unified Sewage Agency, 1998.

Gasser, J. A. Sodium Hypochlorite: The Real Story. *Operations Forum*, 15, 10, 18–22, October 1998.

Seeking Alternatives to Cl_2 Disinfection. *Water Technology News*, August 1998.

CHAPTER 4

Chloramination

Fish gotta swim and birds gotta fly.
But they don't last long if they try. (Tom Lehrer, 1965)

4.1 CHLORAMINATION: A MEETING OF THE MINDS

ON Monday, the DST reconvened. Over the weekend, Nancy Jo had done a considerable amount of research and reading on the topic of chloramination (see Figure 4.1). From her studies, she had come to the conclusion that chloramination was not a viable disinfection alternative for use at the Authority. Several reasons (actually factors) drove her to this conclusion, but the factors were not important at this point. Ensuring that all potential alternative disinfection processes for Rachel's Creek were looked at by her team (the DST) was important. Nancy Jo wanted to ensure that if the DST was going to eliminate any alternative outright, that it was done correctly. Her team would do their homework, discuss it thoroughly, and to eliminate any of the alternatives, they would all come to the same conclusion—a "meeting" of the minds.

4.1.1 THE MEETING

As always, the Safety Director stood before the DST with his flip charts, prepared to write down the team's input:

- Chloramination has been successfully used to disinfect drinking water supplies in the United States and Canada for decades. Denver, Colorado, for instance, has used chloramine since 1917.
- Chloramines are a combination of chlorine and a small amount of ammonia.
- More and more water utilities are switching to chloramines instead

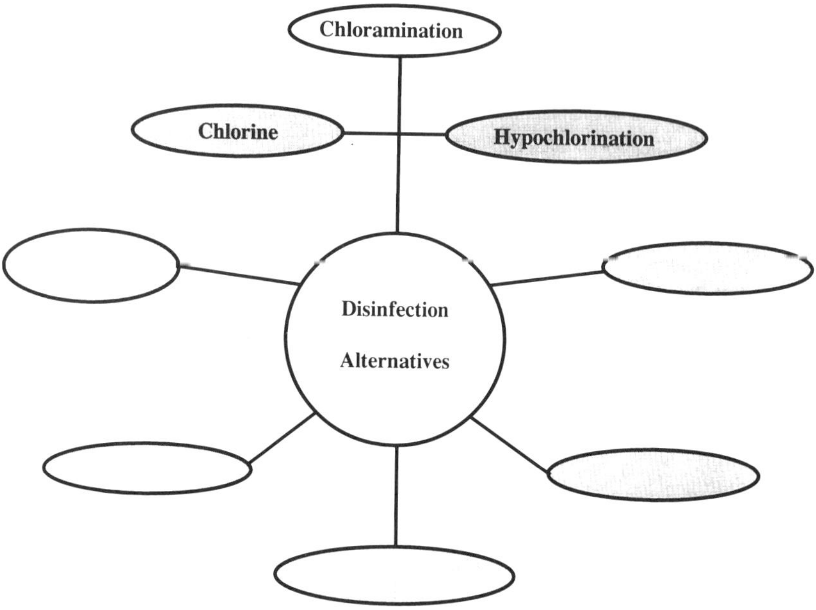

Figure 4.1 Chloramination alternative.

of free chlorine, to cut down on disinfection by-products and thus meet tougher drinking water standards.

- Chloramination of water is performed to produce a more stable disinfectant than free chlorine. Chloramine has been shown to reduce the formation of THMs [trihalomethanes are a suspected carcinogen (cancer-causing agent), created in small amounts as a by-product when natural organics in water combine with chlorine] and other disinfection by-products (DBPs) by as much as 80%, while reducing certain taste and odor problems.
- In some parts of the United States (especially the Midwest and South), as many as one-third to one-half of the utilities serving over 50,000 customers currently practice chloramination. However, at present, chlorine is still most commonly used as the disinfectant of choice because it is quick, effective, safe, and the least expensive method of water disinfection.
- Chlorine is quicker acting than chloramines but is used up faster as it reacts with contaminants in the water. Chlorine also forms chemical compounds called THMs when it mixes with organic compounds. Chloramines are also safe and effective, but react more slowly than chlorine. However, they stay active longer, and they do not form THMs when mixing with organics in water.

- Chloramines do not "affect" the pH of water or wastewater.
- Chloramines are toxic to fish and must be removed from effluent, just as chlorine must be removed (in many cases).
- Chloramines are biocides.
- Like Cl_2, chloramines are oxidants and kill bacteria by penetrating their cell walls and disrupting their metabolism.
- Chloramines do remain as residual.
- As with chlorine, municipalities aim for 1 to 2 mg/L (ppm) chloramine residual in the potable water supply.
- Chloramine is an effective bactericide that produces fewer disinfection by-products than gaseous chlorine; it is generated on-site. Usually, chloramine-forming reactions are 99% complete within a few minutes.
- Chloramine is a weak disinfectant. It is much less effective against viruses or protozoa than free chlorine.
- Chloramine is appropriate for use as a secondary disinfectant to prevent bacterial regrowth in a drinking water distribution system.
- In the chloramination process, chlorine (gaseous solution or sodium hypochlorite) is injected into the supply main, followed immediately by injection of ammonia (gaseous solution or as ammonium hydroxide). Adequate mixing and contact time must be provided. The mix of products produced when water, chlorine, and ammonia are combined depends on the ratio of chlorine to ammonia, and the pH of the water. Chlorine to ammonia ratios of 5:1 should not be exceeded.
- The generation of chloramines requires the same equipment as chlorination (gaseous or aqueous hypochlorination), plus equipment for adding ammonia (gaseous or aqueous).
- Chemicals used to generate chloramine from ammonia and chlorine gas depend on the ammonia-based chemical used. Anhydrous ammonia is the least expensive, whereas ammonium sulfate is the most expensive.
- When ranked by biocidal efficiency (the effectiveness of the disinfectant against a number of viruses and bacteria in the pH range of 6 to 9), chloramine is ranked (best to worst) ozone > chlorine dioxide > free chlorine > chloramines.
- When ranked by stability (reflects a lack of reactivity with constituents other than microorganisms and is a measure of persistence in the treated system), chloramine is ranked (best to worst) chloramines > chlorine dioxide > free chlorine > ozone.
- Chlorine in the form of chloramines is called combined available chlorine.

- The reaction of chlorine with ammonia occurs as follows:

$$NH_3 + HOCl \rightarrow H_2O + NH_2Cl \text{ (monochloramine)}$$

$$NH_2Cl + HOCl \rightarrow H_2O + NHCl_2 \text{ (dichloramine)}$$

$$NHCl_2 + HOCl \rightarrow H_2O + NCl_3 \text{ (trichloramine)}$$

- Organic chloramines cannot be distinguished from other forms of chloramines with standard methods of chloramine analysis.
- Chloramination of wastewater is difficult to control because of the variable concentration of ammonia that may be present in wastewater that has not been fully nitrified during the treatment process. The ammonia concentration is rarely proportionate to the flow rate, thus making flow-paced control an unreliable strategy.

4.2 CHLORAMINATION: THE DISCUSSION

On Tuesday morning, the DST met to discuss their findings on the chloramination alternative and to summarize their recommendations:

Findings:

(1) Chloramination does not have a significant history of use in wastewater treatment.
(2) Gaseous chlorine must be used in the "mix" along with ammonia (both are RMP-regulated substances) to produce chloramines.
(3) No one at the Authority has any experience with chloramination.
(4) Chloramination has a long history of use in treating water supplies. Thus, it could be used at the Authority's two water treatment plants in place of the present elemental chlorine system.

Chloramination parameters fit into the DST matrix as shown in Table 4.1.

Recommendations:

Chloramination is not a suitable disinfectant for use at the Authority for two reasons:

(1) Chloramination requires the use of two RMP substances: chlorine and ammonia. The Authority's flow rates would require stocking and using chlorine and ammonia quantities above the RMP threshold limits; thus, choosing the chloramination alternative for Authority plants would still require us to comply with all RMP compliance requirements.
(2) Our State Water Control Board prohibits chloramination of wastewater and only allows for secondary chloramination of drinking water.

TABLE 4.1. Matrix for Determining the Applicability of Alternative Disinfection Techniques.

Alternative Disinfection Technique (e.g., Cl_2, BrCl, and O_3)	
Consideration	Chloramination
Size of plant	50 MGD (suitable for all levels)
Applicable level of treatment prior to disinfection	All levels
Equipment reliability	?
Process control	?
Relative complexity of technology	Complex
Safety concerns—transportation on-site	Yes, substantial
Bactericidal	Poor
Virucidal	Poor
Fish toxicity	Toxic
Hazardous by-products	Yes
Persistent residual	Very long
Contact time	Long
Contributes D.O.	No
Reacts with ammonia	Yes
Color removal	Moderate
Increased dissolved solids	Yes
pH dependent	Yes
O & M sensitive	Moderate
Corrosive	Yes
Covered by PSM/RMP	Yes

4.3 CHLORAMINATION: THE BOTTOM LINE

Nancy Jo was back on the treadmill, thinking that eliminating the chloramination alternative had been an easy effort—a no-brainer. ". . . Three analyzed, one eliminated, five to go," she told herself. Her mind was working full blast on the next alternative: chlorine dioxide. She had some knowledge of chlorine dioxide and its history as a disinfectant used for treating water/wastewater, but she wanted more information. So, after her exercise session, she was going to attack the 3-foot stack of data-filled documents that sat on her kitchen table. The DST was scheduled to reconvene on Thursday. Tomorrow, Wednesday, was reserved for research and study.

The total number of responses from her survey now stood at 53 and counting.

4.4 REFERENCE

Lehrer, T. *That Was the Year That Was,* Reprise Records R6179, 1965.

CHAPTER 5

Chlorine Dioxide

Pollution, Pollution,
You can use the latest toothpaste,
And then rinse your mouth with industrial waste. (Tom Lehrer, 1965)

5.1 THE CHLORINE DIOXIDE ALTERNATIVE: AN EASY DECISION

NANCY Jo arrived at the conference room early. After having spent a couple of hours last night reviewing information on chlorine dioxide (see Figure 5.1), she felt she was now ready for today's discussion on that topic. She arrived a bit early because she wanted to sit down and look over the schedule for the coming weeks. From the information she examined last night on chlorine dioxide, she realized that the DST would be able to make quick work of this alternative.

Looking at the schedule, she made a few notes and then decided that if the DST finished with chlorine dioxide today, as she expected they would, they would not convene tomorrow (Friday) but instead would convene Monday to discuss the bromine chloride alternative, and before Friday of next week, they should be able to get through both the bromine chloride and the potassium permanganate alternatives. "This will work out well," she told herself, "very well, indeed." With bromine chloride and potassium permanganate out of the way, that would only leave ozone and UV, which she realized might take a bit longer to evaluate than some of the others.

Either way, Nancy Jo's intention was to finish screening all the alternatives within the next two to two and a half weeks. This would allow the DST (and herself) enough time to put together a "dynamite" presentation package for the GM.

Satisfied with her plans, Nancy Jo sat in the boardroom reading about chlorine dioxide until the other DST members arrived.

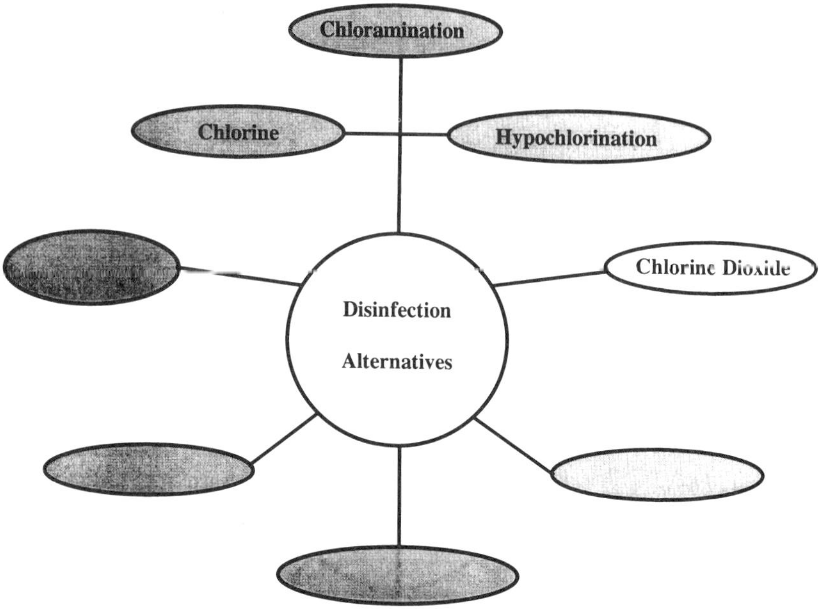

Figure 5.1 Chlorine dioxide alternative.

5.2 CHLORINE DIOXIDE: THE FACTS

The DST Safety Director, felt pen in hand, was ready to record the DST's findings on chlorine dioxide. First, he recorded the following preliminary information on chlorine dioxide.

Sir Humphrey Davy (in 1814) discovered chlorine dioxide as a product of an experiment (a reaction) using potassium chlorate and sulfuric acid. However, it was not used to any extent commercially until around 1940. First used in the pulp and paper industries as a bleaching agent as a replacement for chlorine, eventually it was used in water treatment applications because it is an effective oxidant for eliminating taste and odor problems that occur when free chlorine is contacted with a water that contains phenolic compounds (Bryant et al., 1992).

Initially used in Europe (where industrial discharge of phenols has been a serious concern in contaminating surface water supplies), only recently has interest risen in the United States for its use. This recent interest came about because chlorine dioxide has the advantage of not directly forming halogenated DBPs, which are a concern with the use of free chlorine.

Although chlorine dioxide has been successfully used in the United States for nearly 50 years to disinfect potable water supplies, especially for waters containing phenols or other taste and odor-producing compounds, for color reduction, and for oxidation of inorganic compounds such as iron, manganese, or sulfur compounds (which detract from the aesthetic quality of the water), the USEPA stated in 1986 that no applications of chlorine dioxide disinfection of municipal wastewaters are known at the present time. The only documented use of chlorine dioxide for treating or disinfecting wastewaters is provided by industrial appliers such as refineries, paper and pulp and others, where it has been used successfully to oxidize phenols, mercaptans, cyanides, and many sulfur-containing compounds. It has also had some application in polishing, or as a point source treatment in the plant process. Chlorine dioxide has also been successfully used to treat reclaimed water.

After recording the preliminary information above, the recorder listed the following input from the DST members.

- Chlorine dioxide (ClO_2) is a gas whose color changes from yellowish-green to orangish-red as the concentration in water increases. It condenses to form a red, highly unstable liquid that freezes at −59°C and boils at +11°C.
- Generation of chlorine dioxide generally results from reactions involving either sodium chlorite ($NaClO_2$) or sodium chlorate ($NaClO_3$).
- Generation of chlorine dioxide involving the reaction of sodium chlorite ($NaClO_2$) with chlorine to produce gaseous chlorine dioxide occurs according to the following reaction (produced in a ratio of 1 mole of chlorine to 2 moles of chlorite): $2NaClO_2 + Cl_2 \rightarrow 2ClO_2 + 2NaCl$.
- Sodium chlorite is much more expensive than gaseous chlorine per unit weight expressed as chlorine.
- Chlorine dioxide is a proven bactericide equal to or greater than chlorine in disinfecting power and has a higher oxidation potential.
- Because chlorine dioxide gas is sensitive to pressure and temperature, it cannot be shipped in bulk. Therefore, it must be generated and used on-site.
- Chlorine dioxide is an unstable and explosive gas and for this reason must be generated on-site.
- Through experience we know that chlorine dioxide gas can be handled safely by dilution with sufficient air or nitrogen to keep the chlorine dioxide concentration below 10%.
- An advantage in using chlorine dioxide is that it does not react with ammonia to form the potentially toxic chloramines.
- Chlorine dioxide is active in water for at least 48 hours as a bactericide, and it may have a longer period of effectiveness than that of chlorine.
- A summary of the effect of chlorine dioxide on various drinking water components is shown in Table 5.1.

TABLE 5.1. Summary of the Effect of Chlorine Dioxide on Drinking Water Components.

Constituent	Reaction
Selected natural and synthetic organics	Can react to form chlorite
Iron and manganese	Oxidized
Color	Removed
THMs	Lowered
Organics	Oxidized
Phenols	Reacts to form chlorinated phenols and quinones

- The greater efficacy of chlorine dioxide compared with chlorine, notably at higher pH, points to an increase in use for disinfection purposes (in water treatment and industrial waste applications).
- Because chlorine dioxide is a more potent "microbiocide" than chlorine, microbial risk is not increased as long as adequate levels of the disinfectant are used.
- Because it is a more potent or "efficacious" agent, lower levels of chlorine dioxide can be used to get the same effective inactivation of microbes.
- Chlorine dioxide has been found to be active against pathogens that are resistant to chlorine.
- Chlorine dioxide's oxidizing and disinfecting properties remain constant over the wide pH range of 4 to 10. This is different from the active forms of chlorine, which are strongly affected by the pH. A comparison of these factors with various disinfectants is shown in Table 5.2.
- One of the commonly used methods of generating chlorine dioxide is shown in Figure 5.2. This system involves the dissolution of

TABLE 5.2. Biochemical Efficiency, Stability, and the Effects of pH on Efficiency of Some Disinfectants.

Disinfectant	Biocidal*	Stability*	Effect of the pH Efficiency (pH = 6–9)
Ozone	1	4	Little influence
Chlorine dioxide	2	3	Efficiency slightly increases with the increase of pH
Chlorine	3	2	Efficiency decreases considerably with the increase of pH
Chloramines	4	1	Little influence

*The indicated characteristics decrease from 1 to 4 (1 is maximum, 4 the minimum).

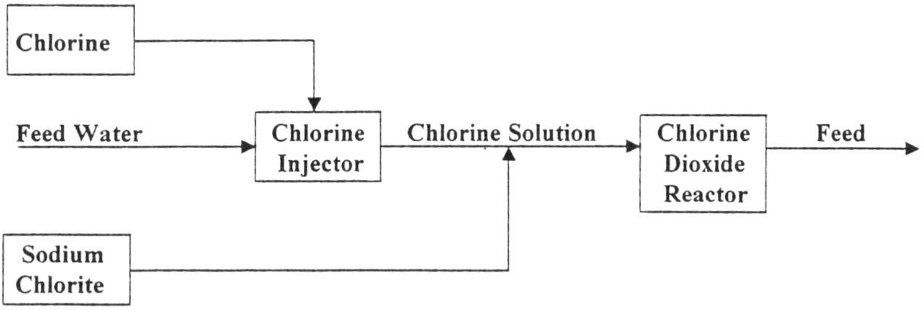

Figure 5.2 Basic chlorine dioxide system (chlorine/chlorite solution).

chlorine into a feed water stream, followed by subsequent contact with a sodium chlorite stream in reactor or generator. The two streams are mixed for reaction, either within the reactor or in the reactor influent pipeline (Figure 5.2). Acid can be added if necessary for controlling the reaction within the optimum pH range for chlorine dioxide generation (Bryant et al., 1992).

- The environmental impacts associated with chlorine dioxide use as a wastewater disinfectant have not been well established.
- Chlorine dioxide has not received a great deal of attention as a wastewater disinfectant because of its on-site generation requirements and high chemical costs.
- The overall chlorine dioxide system is relatively complex to operate and maintain compared with chlorination.
- Although chlorine dioxide has been shown to be an effective wastewater disinfectant, few pilot studies have been done, and experience is quite limited in the United States.

5.3 CHLORINE DIOXIDE: THE DISCUSSION

After lunch, the DST reconvened and put together their list of findings and recommendations on chlorine dioxide:

Findings:

(1) Chlorine dioxide does not have a significant history of use in the treatment of municipal wastewater.
(2) Chlorine dioxide must be generated on-site and is much more expensive than elemental chlorine.
(3) Chlorine dioxide has several safety-related problems; it is dangerous because two dangerous gases (chlorine and sodium chlorite) must be handled.
(4) Its use will not preclude the Authority from having to comply with RMP

TABLE 5.2. Matrix for Determining the Applicability of Alternative Disinfection Techniques.

Alternative Disinfection Technique (e.g., Cl_2, BrCl, and O_3)	
Consideration	Chlorine Dioxide
Size of plant	50 MGD (suitable for small to medium-sized plants)
Applicable level of treatment prior to disinfection	Secondary
Equipment reliability	?
Process control	No experience
Relative complexity of technology	Moderate
Safety concerns—transportation on-site	Yes, substantial
Bactericidal	Good
Virucidal	Good
Fish toxicity	Toxic
Hazardous by-products	Yes
Persistent residual	Moderate
Contact time	Moderate to long
Contributes D.O.	No
Reacts with ammonia	No
Color removal	Yes
Increased dissolved solids	Yes
pH dependent	No
O & M sensitive	?
Corrosive	Yes
Covered by PSM/RMP	Yes

Source: USEPA, 1986.

because we will still have to store, use, and handle chlorine at levels above the threshold limit.

(5) No one at the Authority has any experience using chlorine dioxide.

Chlorine dioxide parameters fit into the DST matrix (see Table 5.3).

Recommendations: Chlorine dioxide is not a "proven" disinfectant alternative for wastewater treatment. Furthermore, from the data contained in the matrix, the use of chlorine dioxide is obviously not a viable disinfection alternative for use at Rachel's Creek (or anywhere else at the Authority).

5.4 CHLORINE DIOXIDE: THE BOTTOM LINE

Back on the treadmill, Nancy Jo was running along at a moderate pace and thinking about the day's events. By the close of business today, the DST had eliminated chlorine dioxide from further consideration as a disinfection alternative for Rachel's Creek. "Wasn't all that difficult to do," she told herself. "No one else I know of is using it . . . and besides, chlorine dioxide does not remove us from EPA's RMP regulatory umbrella."

Shifting speed on the treadmill to increase the pace, she also shifted her train of thought. Actually, her mind was thinking along two lines: First, she had told the DST to reconvene on Monday (that would give them the weekend—enough time to study bromine chloride), and she figured they would be able to come up with a finding on bromine chloride by no later than noon Tuesday, which would give them time to prepare for a discussion of potassium permanganate on Wednesday and finish with it by the end of the week.

The other train of thought she was engaged in was about the "other" Authority plants—those other POTWs using chlorine for chlorination and sulfur dioxide for dechlorination, and the two water treatment plants currently using chlorine for disinfection. Nancy Jo realized that when she presented the DST's findings to the GM, that her "dynamite" presentation could end up exploding in her face if she did not factor in everything. The everything being, "OK," the GM would say, "you have decided that substitution of chlorine is required and have recommended your alternative selection will get us off the hook with the regulators . . . that RMP thing . . . so what are we going to do about the other Authority plants using chlorine and other covered substances at present?"

This is the question (at least one of them anyway) that she was absolutely certain the GM would ask. As she speeded up the treadmill and her pace to accompany it, she told herself emphatically: "Well, whatever he asks, I will have the answer . . . and that is that!"

The survey forms were still coming in; total number of respondents to date: 101 and counting.

5.5 REFERENCES

Bryant, E. A. et al. *Disinfection Alternatives for Safe Drinking Water.* New York: Van Nostrand Reinhold, 1992.

Lehrer, T. *That Was the Year That Was,* Reprise Records R6179, 1965.

USEPA. *Design Manual: Municipal Wastewater Disinfection*, 1986.

CHAPTER 6

Bromine Chloride

Lots of things there that you can drink,
But stay away from the kitchen sink,
The breakfast garbage that you throw into the Bay,
They drink for lunch in San Jose. (Tom Lehrer, 1965)

6.1 MORNING PRELUDE

WE have all heard the saying "different strokes for different folks." This phrase certainly fit Nancy Jo to a T in more ways than we can count. After pushing the treadmill through a torturous routine each evening, Nancy Jo would clean up, put in a couple of hours on homework from work, and then read for a couple of hours. She'd sleep until 4:00 A.M. and then jump out of bed, do the teeth, hair, makeup, get dressed. Then she would either remain in her condo reading work-related materials until time to go to work, or she'd go in and do her reading there.

Having completed her standard early morning routine, Nancy Jo opted for her office at work this morning, because she had left two excellent articles about bromine chloride on her desk. She wanted to study them before the DST session began.

About an hour later, Nancy Jo finished reading the articles (sometimes she read slowly, highlighting and absorbing key information and then transferring the highlights to written notes. These articles deserved that level of her attention). The articles: Scott F. Biondi's *Wastewater Disinfection Alternative—Bromine Chloride* (1991) and Forbes and Trainque's "Implementation of a Bromine Based CSO [Combined Sewer Overflows] Disinfection System for Burlington, Vermont" (1992)—both excellent, informative articles—were exactly what she had been looking for.

At eight o'clock the DST reconvened and began the day's business: bromine chloride.

6.2 BROMINE CHLORIDE: PERTINENT FACTS

The Safety Director recorded the following introductory information on the next disinfection alternative: bromine chloride (see Figure 6.1).

Bromine chloride is a mixture of bromine and chlorine. It forms hydrocarbons and hydrochloric acid when mixed with water. Bromine chloride is an excellent disinfectant that reacts quickly and does not normally produce any long-term residuals.

The reactions that occur when bromine chloride is added to the wastewater are similar to those that occur when chlorine is added. The major difference is the production of bromamine compounds rather than chloramines. Bromamine compounds are excellent disinfectants but are less stable than chloramines, and they dissipate quickly. In most cases, the bromamines decay into less toxic compounds rapidly and are undetectable in the plant effluent.

The factors that affect performance are similar to those affecting the performance of the chlorine disinfection process. Factors including effluent quality and contact time have a direct impact on the performance of the process.

With the introductory information on bromine chloride (BrCl) duly recorded, the DST shifted to recording the facts they had obtained. These facts are listed as follows:

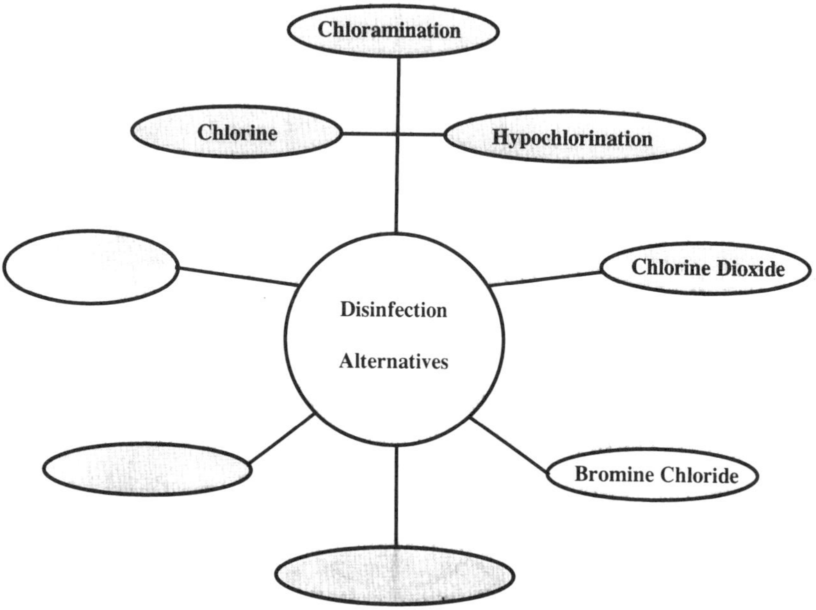

Figure 6.1 Bromine chloride alternative.

- BrCl is approved by USEPA as a disinfectant for wastewater treatment.
- Bromine chloride is manufactured from bromine and chlorine.
- When added to water, BrCl hydrolyzes to hypobromous acid (HOBr) very rapidly and forms monobromamines and diabromamines when added to water containing ammonia-nitrogen.
- Bromine chloride has a sharp, harsh, penetrating odor.
- In both the liquid and vapor phases BrCl is a strong, oxidizing agent.
- Bromine chloride is classified as an interhalogen compound because it is formed from two different halogens.
- At equilibrium, bromine chloride is a fuming dark-red liquid below 5°C.
- It can be withdrawn either as a liquid from storage vessels equipped with dip tubes under its own pressure or as a vapor from equipment similar to that used for chlorine.
- Bromine chloride is effective at higher pH levels.
- Bromine chloride can be applied at lower dosages than chlorine to effect the same pathogen kill.
- Bromine chloride is a hazardous and corrosive chemical and requires special transportation, handling, storage, and use precautions; it is an extremely corrosive compound in the presence of low concentrations of moisture.
- Like chlorine and bromine, bromine chloride may be stored in steel containers.
- Bromine chloride has a higher density than chlorine; its specific gravity is 2.34 compared to 1.47 for chlorine.
- Bromine chloride is a more effective and less toxic disinfectant than chlorine; lack of proven experience at large scale plants makes it unsuitable for application at most POTWs.
- Contact time is less than for chlorine, so contact chambers are smaller (see Figure 6.2).
- When in contact with skin and other tissues, liquid BrCl causes severe burns. Low concentrations of the vapor are extremely irritating to the eyes and respiratory tract.
- Bromine chloride is subject to reliquefaction, which causes dissociation of the vapor, defeating its purpose.
- Because BrCl is classified as a corrosive liquid and not a hazardous gas, it is easy to transport, store, and handle.
- A specially designed feeder system has been developed to safely and efficiently apply liquid BrCl (see Figure 6.2). In field-scale applications, problems with the liquid feed equipment have occurred.
- Environmental impacts associated with bromine chloride disinfection are less adverse than those associated with chlorine.

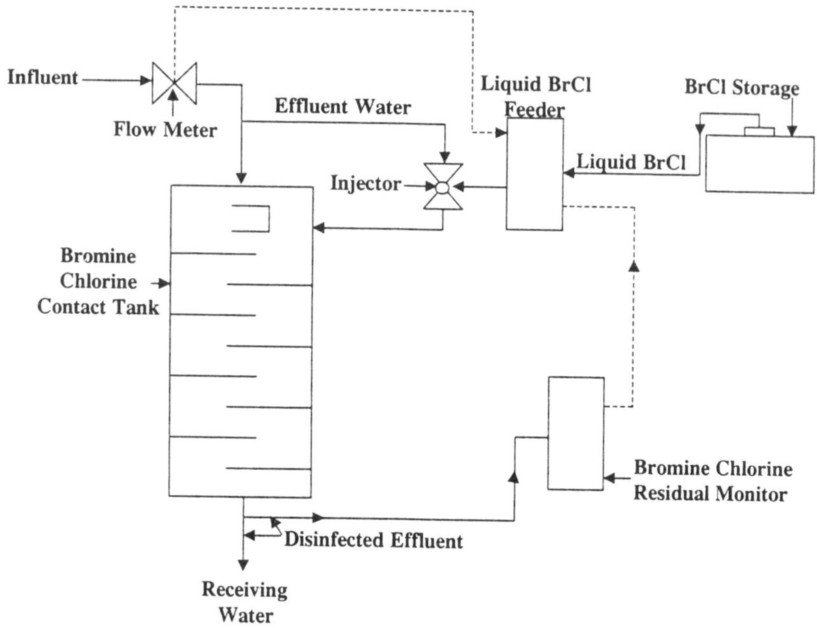

Figure 6.2 Bromine chloride feeder system. *Source:* Adaptation from Metcalf & Eddy, p. 508, 1991.

6.3 BROMINE CHLORIDE: THE DISCUSSION

This session took only about 2 hours to complete. Because of the short amount of time involved, the DST decided to finalize their findings prior to lunch, so that the members would have time in the afternoon to catch up on other work-related matters.

The DST recorded the following findings on bromine chloride:

Findings:

(1) Bromine chloride is a proven disinfectant with a significant bacteriocidal effectiveness over a broad range of pathogens (such as viruses, cysts, and certain bacteria).
(2) Disinfection with bromine chloride requires lower dosages than chlorine to achieve pathogen kill.
(3) Use of bromine chloride raises some serious safety concerns.

Bromine chloride parameters fit into the DST matrix (see Table 6.1).

Recommendations: Bromine chloride's use for wastewater disinfection is relatively new, and a good database and track record are presently not available (USEPA, 1986). It is a toxic, highly corrosive chemical that requires special handling and safety precautions. Because of no readily available local supply and the technical difficulties associated with the use of bromine chloride, we do not consider it a feasible choice for disinfecting flows at Rachel's Creek. Because of safety concerns relative to bromine chloride and the fact that Rachel's Creek WWTP is located near the downtown waterfront area, we also do not recommend it for use by the Authority at our other facilities.

6.4 BROMINE CHLORIDE: THE BOTTOM LINE

Having finished her workout on the treadmill, taken a hot bath, and finished eating a light salad, Nancy Jo sat on her living room couch and reviewed the day's events. Even though the DST had eliminated bromine chloride from further consideration as a disinfection alternative for use at Rachel's Creek and at the Authority, Nancy Jo wanted to make sure that they hadn't overlooked anything.

Later, satisfied with the DST's progress to date, Nancy Jo's thoughts shifted to potassium permanganate. After about an hour of reading on the subject, she was pretty much convinced that the DST would make quick

TABLE 6.1. Matrix for Determining the Applicability of Alternative Disinfection Techniques.

Alternative Disinfection Technique (e.g., Cl_2, BrCl, and O_3)	
Consideration	Bromine Chloride
Size of plant	All sizes
Applicable level of treatment prior to disinfection	Secondary
Equipment reliability	?
Process control	Problematic
Relative complexity of technology	Moderate
Safety concerns—transportation on-site	Yes, substantial
Bactericidal	Good
Virucidal	Fair to poor
Fish toxicity	Slight to moderate
Hazardous by-products	Yes
Persistent residual	Short
Contact time	Moderate
Contributes D.O.	No
Reacts with ammonia	Yes
Color removal	?
Increased dissolved solids	Yes
pH dependent	Yes
O & M sensitive	Moderate
Corrosive	Yes
Covered by PSM/RMP	Yes (bromine)

work of potassium permanganate. Then the focus would shift to ozone—a much more detailed subject area because ozone has a considerable history of use in wastewater treatment for disinfection purposes. At this point she wasn't sure if they would launch right into a study of ozone after finishing with potassium permanganate, or if they would wait a while to take some time to thoroughly study the ozone alternative. "Oh, well . . . I'll get it all figured out," she told herself, as she put the disinfection study material away.

The survey forms were still coming in; total number of respondents to date: 109 and counting.

6.5 REFERENCES

Biondi, S. F. *Wastewater Disinfection Alternative—Bromine Chloride. Oper. Forum*, 8, 6, 20–23, 1991.

Forbes, E. J. and Trainque, M. A. Implementation of a Bromine Based CSO Disinfection System for Burlington, Vermont. Paper presented at *Water Environ. Fed. 65th Annu. Conf. and Exposition,* New Orleans, Louisiana, 449–460, 1992.

Lehrer, T. *That Was the Year That Was*. Reprise Records R6179, 1965.

Metcalf and Eddy. *Wastewater Engineering: Treatment, Disposal, Reuse* (3rd ed.). New York: McGraw-Hill, Inc., 1991.

USEPA. *Design Manual: Municipal Wastewater Disinfection*, 1986.

CHAPTER 7

Potassium Permanganate

So go to the city, see the crazy people there.
Like lambs to the slaughter,
They're drinking the water . . . (Tom Lehrer, 1965)

7.1 POTASSIUM PERMANGANATE: QUICK WORK

NANCY Jo sat in her office reading and taking notes. She now felt that she had enough information about today's topic: potassium permanganate. About an hour earlier, she had finished reading an article "Potassium Permanganate," in Bryant (et al.) *Disinfection Alternatives for Safe Drinking Water* (1992) by Ficek and Reidies—"A really good book . . . and definitely a good article . . . a good discussion on potassium permanganate."

From Ficek and Reidies' work, Nancy Jo could clearly see that the DST would have little difficulty in eliminating potassium permanganate as a disinfection alternative for Rachel's Creek and/or the Authority. According to Ficek and Reidies, "Potassium permanganate is a widely used chemical oxidizing agent throughout the ['water industry']. While generally not considered for a disinfecting role, it can still have an important effect on the development of a disinfecting strategy by serving as an alternative to chlorine or other disinfecting chemicals at locations in a plant where chemical oxidation is a primary goal" (p. 259).

Obviously, potassium permanganate has some application for disinfecting drinking water, but seems to have little to do with wastewater disinfection.

Over the next hour or so, after reading various other sources, she was able to confirm to her own satisfaction that potassium permanganate doesn't have that much at all to do with disinfecting wastewater, municipal wastewater that is. According to Vella (1996), in a paper presented in New Orleans at the American Institute of Chemical Engineer's (AIChE) Spring Meeting, ". . . potassium permanganate is a strong oxidizing agent that may be used in aqueous solution over a wide pH range. It has been successfully used for the treatment of sulfur compounds, phonemics, and other organic materials

. . . potassium permanganate [can be used] for pretreatment of industrial wastewaters containing phenolics and inorganic sulfur compounds."

"So, it does have application for use in treating some industrial wastestreams," she told herself. "The question is: Why does the GM want us (the DST) to even consider it for use in treating municipal wastewater at Rachel's Creek?" She didn't know why. However, she was reasonably sure at this point (unless shown contradictory information by the DST members) that the DST would make quick work of potassium permanganate.

7.2 POTASSIUM PERMANGANATE: GOING THROUGH THE MOTIONS

Convinced that potassium permanganate (see Figure 7.1), although perhaps useful for treating drinking water, was not a viable disinfection alternative for use at Rachel's Creek or anywhere else in the Authority, Nancy Jo wasted little time in bringing the DST meeting to order. She wanted to move forward as quickly as possible with their analysis, recommendations, and final decision regarding potassium permanganate, so they could move on to "bigger and better" things. She asked the Safety Director to take up his recorder's station, and opened the discussion. He recorded the following background information first.

Potassium permanganate ($KMnO_4$) is an oxidant (primarily used in water treatment) that was first used in the early 1900s in London. Widespread use

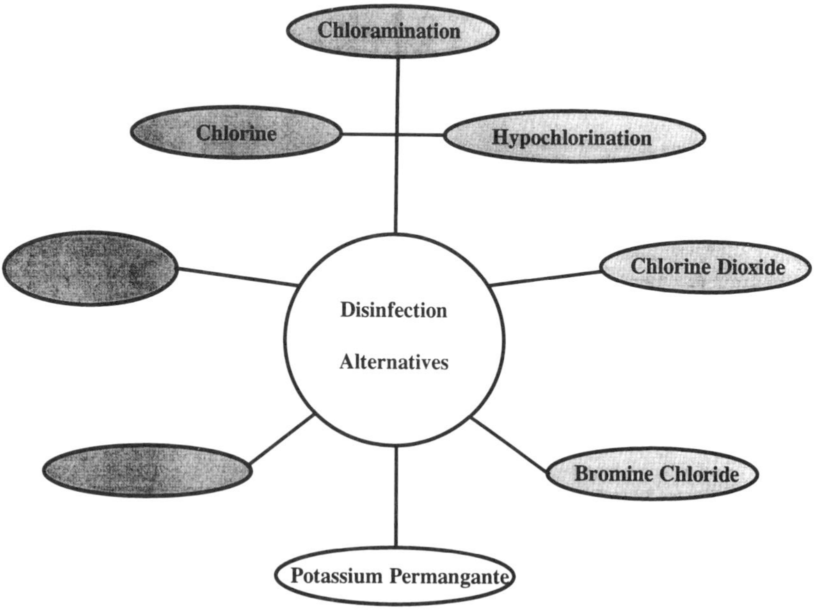

Figure 7.1 Potassium permanganate alternative.

of potassium permanganate, however, did not occur until the 1960s, when its effectiveness for controlling tastes and odors was recognized. Potassium permanganate has also been used in wastewater treatment (primarily in treatment of industrial wastewater) on a limited basis; it is not widely accepted as a disinfection alternative for municipal wastewater treatment.

7.3 POTASSIUM PERMANGANATE: PERTINENT FACTS

From input provided by DST members, the recorder listed the following information on potassium permanganate.

- Potassium permanganate is commercially available in crystalline form in a variety of grades and package sizes.
- The Department of Transportation classifies potassium permanganate as an oxidizer, requiring it to be labeled as such in shipping containers.
- Potassium permanganate occurs in the form of deep purple (almost black) crystals that, when added to water, turn the water purple until it finally dissipates after the completion of the oxidizing action.
- Concentrations as low as 0.05 ppm may still have some noticeable color. For this reason and to allow completion of the oxidizing reaction, it should be fed as early in the treatment process as possible.
- The solubility of potassium permanganate is strongly temperature dependent.
- The solution rate depends on temperature, particle size, agitation, and the concentration of other salts already in solution.
- Technical grades of potassium permanganate crystals have a tendency to cake together, especially under high-humidity conditions.
- Potassium permanganate is highly reactive, and nearly all of the chemical reactions release heat (are exothermic).
- Potassium permanganate is effective against a wide range of microorganisms: bacteria, fungi, viruses, and algae.
- Potassium permanganate is more effective than chlorine in controlling many taste- and odor-causing substances in raw water.
- Industrywide experience (in water treatment) has shown that potassium permanganate is effective in controlling THMs.
- Potassium permanganate is not registered with the USEPA as a disinfectant.

7.4 POTASSIUM PERMANGANATE: THE DISCUSSION

The last item listed was the focus of the DST's discussion on the merits of selecting or not selecting potassium permanganate as a possible disinfection alternative for Rachel's Creek WWTP. It was a short discussion. None of the members had found any efficacy of potassium permanganate as a disinfectant, let alone any related to its possible use at Rachel's Creek. That potassium permanganate is not EPA registered meant that it could not be seriously considered as a viable alternative. Because it already fell far short of fitting into the matrix, taking the effort to make it fit was futile. For these reasons, the DST decided to drop it from further consideration.

7.5 ON THE TREADMILL

Running along at a rapid pace on her treadmill, Nancy Jo was thinking through the day's events. In the DST's discussion regarding potassium permanganate, she realized that they had not given this topic the same amount or level of detail as they had the previous disinfection alternatives. However, she had little difficulty in justifying their modus operandi, because potassium permanganate simply did not provide the same beneficial uses as some of the earlier alternatives and definitely did not meet the criteria to replace elemental chlorine.

However, they had gone through the motions in evaluating potassium permanganate as a possible alternative disinfectant; they had stuck to their guiding principle of evaluating each alternative on a case-by-case basis. The obvious lack of state-of-the-art design information, lack of local expertise, and the failure of USEPA to even consider potassium permanganate as a viable disinfection alternative had all worked to seal its fate.

Before the DST had adjourned for the day, Nancy Jo had laid out the agenda and timeline for evaluating the last two alternatives: ozone and UV disinfection. Having full knowledge that both of these processes were legitimate disinfection alternatives for substitution of elemental chlorine, she directed the DST to spend the rest of the week researching ozone. They were to reconvene on Monday to discuss ozone and to finish by Thursday so that they would have a little time to do research on UV, which they were scheduled to discuss the following Monday.

This was the plan; Nancy Jo had little doubt that they would be successful in finishing their preliminary study in no more than 2 weeks. This would allow enough time to put together their findings and present them to the GM.

The survey forms were rolling in; total number of respondents to date: 123 and counting.

7.6 REFERENCES

Ficek, K. J. and Reidies, A. H. in Bryant et al. *Disinfection Alternatives for Safe Drinking Water*. New York: Van Nostrand Reinhold, 1992.

Lehrer, T., *That Was the Year That Was*. Reprise Records R6179, 1965.

Vella, P.A. Potassium Permanganate Pretreatment of Industrial Wastewater. Paper presented at the *Spring Meeting, New Orleans, Louisiana: AIChE,* February 26, 1996.

CHAPTER 8

Ozone

The environmentalists are right about one thing: Dirty water kills. Millions of people are dying needlessly all over the world because of it. But are the main culprits man-made pollution and chlorinated chemicals? Try endemic poverty, bad plumbing and lack of access to basic water chlorination techniques. Every year, nearly 1.5 billion people—mostly children under five—suffer from preventable water-borne diseases such as cholera, typhoid fever, amoebic dysentery, bacterial gastroenteritis, giardiasis, schistosomiasis, and various viral diseases such as hepatitis A. Yet now there is a mounting campaign, led by environmental activists in wealthy industrialized nations, to eliminate every last man-made chlorine molecule from the face of the earth. (Malkin and Fumento)

8.1 OZONE: PRELUDE

IF you mentioned ozone to the average person, the first thought that might come to mind is the ozone hole. Another person might associate the word ozone with the ozone shield. Another (more rare) individual might associate ozone with its chemical properties.

At the moment, Nancy Jo, after having completed an intense workout on the treadmill, a soothing hot bath, and the hated but mandatory requirement to feed herself, sat at the desk in her home office, sorting through the maze of paper, articles, journals, technical manuals, P&Ids (piping and instrumentation diagrams), trying to glean as much information about ozone (i.e., O_3) as she could.

It was Sunday evening, late—very late. The previous week had gone by quickly. After the DST had made quick work of potassium permanganate on Monday, they returned to their normal work stations to catch up on their normal workloads (and to study ozone, of course) and finish off the week. Of course, in Nancy Jo's case, her current normal workload (her only workload at present) was to come up with a final disinfection alternative's presentation for the GM and to sell him on the DST's final selection, whatever it turned out to be.

"Tomorrow we will attack ozone," she told herself. "It'll take some time, though O_3 is definitely more complicated than a few of the others were, and it does seem to have some history for use in disinfecting wastewater effluent." A few minutes later, she stacked her reference material into a tall, neat pile and pushed it aside. Thirty minutes later, she was in bed. Asleep? Not hardly. When you have microchips for brain cells operating in megabytes going fast-forward, sleep is a requirement, a nuisance and nothing more. Instead, she was thinking about ozone, in a kind of free association: ozone holes, the ozone shield, tropospheric and stratospheric ozone, but mostly, she was just thinking ahead toward making her presentation to the GM.

Then she tossed and turned a bit. Now she was really wide awake, suddenly overwhelmed at how utterly simple the task of water treatment could be. "Disinfection can really be simple," she thought.

What Nancy Jo was thinking about was some of the information in the material she had read earlier in the evening. One report had made the profound statement, "Disinfection is easy, just boil the water before you use it." Now she was almost giggling. "Just boil the water; I wish it was that simple for us," she said aloud.

Then she thought about a simple purification process she had read about in a UNICEF report by American University of Beirut (1984): *Solar Disinfection of Drinking Water and Oral Rehydration Solutions*.

"The following instructions are intended primarily for the benefit of housewives in rural areas in developing countries where safe community water supplies are not available. It is assumed that in these areas waterborne diseases are endemic or sporadic."

Then, instead of counting sheep she recounted the step-by-step procedures on how to disinfect water using solar power and finally, she slept.

8.2 OZONE: BACKGROUND INFORMATION

Before dismissing the DST on the preceding Monday, Nancy Jo asked the Safety Director to prepare a brief introduction (background information) about ozone and ozonation as it applies to wastewater treatment. She had requested that this information be both in writing (for the record, of course) and presented orally by the Safety Director to the DST.

The Safety Director presented the following information on ozone and ozonation to the DST.

The ozone disinfection alternative (see Figure 8.1) is clearly playing an increasing role in water treatment facilities, including residential systems, as an effective disinfectant and oxidizer. Ozone has also been used in disinfecting wastewater effluent and in some regards is growing in usage, at

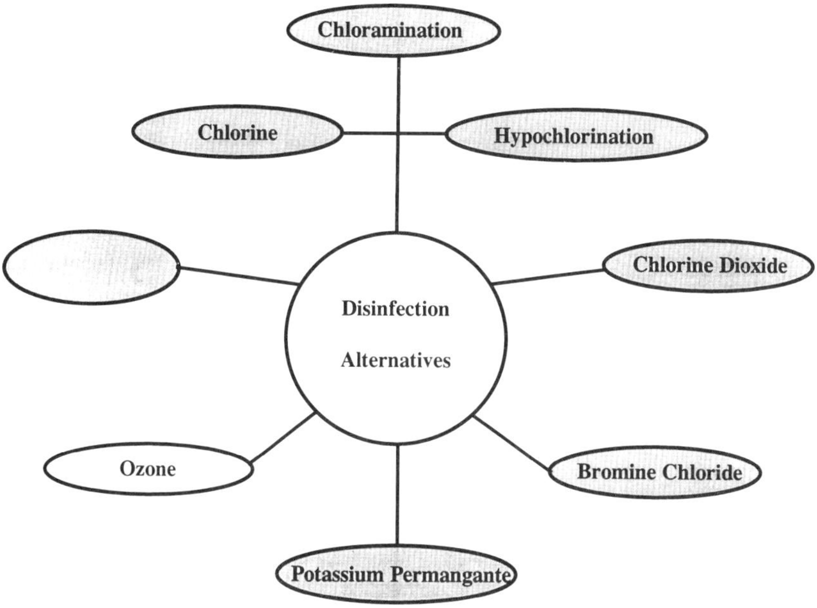

Figure 8.1 Ozone alternative.

least in the testing phase via pilot studies. In some areas, ozone is actually the preferred form of disinfectant. It has the highest oxidation potential, acting quickly to kill any unwanted bacteria or viruses. It also results in no THMs.

According to USEPA (1986), the first U.S. wastewater plant to use ozone for disinfection was Indiantown, Florida, which began operation in 1975. By 1980, about 10 wastewater treatment plants using ozone for disinfection had been constructed. (*Note:* By 1982 this number had increased to 42 POTWs.) Unfortunately, some of these earlier ozone disinfection facilities have chosen to abandon ozone disinfection for one or more of the following reasons: excessive high cost of operation, equipment problems, excessive maintenance cost, and/or inability to attain performance objectives without major modifications. Current regulations for domestic treatment systems limit use of ozonation to filtered effluents, unless the system's effectiveness can be demonstrated prior to installation.

What is ozone? In a nutshell, ozone is an allotrope of oxygen having three atoms to each molecule. It is a powerful oxidizing and disinfecting agent. Formed by passing dry air through a system of high-voltage electrodes, the oxygen in the air is dissociated by the impact of electrons from the discharge electrode. The atomic oxygen then combines with atmospheric oxygen to form ozone in the following reaction: $O + O_2 \rightarrow O_3$. Ozonation is the process whereby ozone is generated and then mixed with the effluent in a contact chamber.

Requiring shorter contact time and dosage than chlorine, ozone is widely used as a primary disinfectant in many parts of the world, but it is relatively new in the United States. Ozone does not directly produce halogenated organic materials unless a bromide ion is present.

Ozone gas is unstable and must be generated on-site. The application of ozone disinfection at Rachel's Creek would be a difficult and costly undertaking. Probably the most cost-effective way to generate the ozone necessary for disinfection would be through the use of an oxygen-fed ozone generator. A secondary disinfectant (usually chlorine) is required, because ozone does not maintain an adequate residual in water.

8.3 OZONE: JUST THE FACTS, MA'AM

After the Safety Director's presentation of the introductory information, the DST members began talking among themselves. Finally, the prospective plant manager addressed Nancy Jo and said: "Seems quite obvious to all of us that ozone is not an alternative for us to spend much time on; we seem to all agree that we should make quick work of it. What do you think, ma'am?"

Nancy Jo had, long ago, come to the same conclusion as the plant manager and the rest of her team had, but she was determined to see each alternative through to its natural end. She said, "I couldn't agree with you more. Ozone won't cut it for us, no doubt about that. So, what I think we should do is go through the drill with this one to make sure we have everything we need in our written report for the Big Guy, then move on to UV."

The DST, in chorus, agreed. The Safety Director, standing at his clean slate concurred.

8.4 OZONE: THE FACTS

- According to Rosen (1976), the advantages of ozonation systems include:
  (1) Few safety problems associated with transportation and storage
  (2) Excellent virucidal and bactericidal properties
  (3) Shorter feasible treatment times (approximately 10 minutes for ozone compared to 30 to 45 minutes with chlorine)
  (4) Improvement of receiving stream quality resulting from high dissolved oxygen concentration of ozone-disinfected effluent
  (5) No increase of total dissolved solids in ozone-treated water

(6) Wastewater quality improvements (including effluent color, odor, and turbidity reductions)

(7) Easy extension of ozone to tertiary polishing

- Ozone (O_3) is an unstable gas produced when oxygen molecules are dissociated into atomic oxygen and subsequently collide with another oxygen molecule.
- The factors that affect ozone's disinfection efficacy include the following (Bell and Smith, 1982; Caverson et al., 1986; Given and Smith, 1979; and Venosa et al., 1980):

  (1) Ozone dose

  (2) Contact time

  (3) Suspended solids

  (4) pH

  (5) Chemical oxygen demand (COD)

  (6) Organic carbon

  (7) Temperature

  (8) Contactor design

- The energy source for dissociating the oxygen molecule can be produced commercially or can occur naturally.
- Some natural sources for ozone production are ultraviolet (UV) light from the sun and lightning during a thunderstorm.
- As a strong oxidizing gas, ozone is both an effective disinfectant and an oxidant of taste and odor compounds.
- Ozone works rapidly to inactivate microorganisms.
- Unlike chlorine, which reacts with water to produce disinfecting species, ozone decomposes in water to produce oxygen and free hydroxyl radicals.
- Effluent quality is the key performance factor for ozonation.
- Operation is particularly important with respect to ozonation systems. Ozone generation is electrical power intensive; therefore, optimization of the system can significantly reduce operating costs (Rakness et al., 1994).
- A common application for oxygen-fed ozone disinfection is in conjunction with an oxygen activated sludge process where the oxygen is reused. Only about 10% of the oxygen in the feed-gas is "used up" in the ozone process; thus, 90% or more is available for the biological treatment process.
- Ozone is an extremely toxic substance. Concentrations in air should not exceed 0.1 ppm. It also has the potential to create an explosive atmosphere. Sufficient ventilation and purging capabilities should be provided.

- Ozone has certain advantages over chlorine for disinfection of wastewater:
  (1) Ozone increases D.O. in the effluent.
  (2) Ozone has a briefer contact time.
  (3) Ozone has no undesirable effects on marine organisms.
  (4) Ozone decreases turbidity and color.
- pH can be an important factor in ozone disinfection.
- In practice, ozone is rarely applied solely for disinfection (in wastewater processing) because of the high cost relative to chlorine and the absence of a disinfecting residual (Hammer and Hammer, p. 260, 1996)
- Ozone decays spontaneously to oxygen, hence its production at locations remote from the point of use is impractical (McGhee, p. 236, 1991).

8.5 OZONATION SYSTEM

Typically, an ozonation system consists of (1) air preparation or oxygen feed, (2) electric power supply, (3) ozone generation, (4) ozone contacting, and (5) ozone contactor exhaust gas destruction. To prevent fouling of the ozone production tubes and to reduce corrosion, ambient air is first dried. Some systems use desiccant dryers in conjunction with compression and refrigerant dryers. To control the rate of ozone production, the voltage or frequency of the electrical supply is varied.

8.6 OZONE: PROCESS FLOW SCHEME

The DST shifted its discussion of ozone/ozonation from the facts to the disinfection process itself. The DST recorder recorded the following information.

As USEPA (1986) points out, the ozone disinfection process consists of a liquid and a gas flow scheme (see Figure 8.2). The feed-gas is typically air or high-purity oxygen. A small percentage (1% wt in air to 4% wt in oxygen) of the feed-gas is converted to ozone within the ozone generator. The ozone containing feed-gas is directed to a contact basin, where it combines with the wastewater. Typically, a high percentage of the ozone, but only a small percentage of the total feed-gas flow, is transferred to the liquid in the contact basin. The disinfection action proceeds in the contact basin. As shown in Figure 8.2, the gas and liquid flows separate after the contact basin. The off-gas is treated to remove the unreacted ozone and is reused, recycled, or discharged to the atmosphere. The disinfected wastewater is discharged to

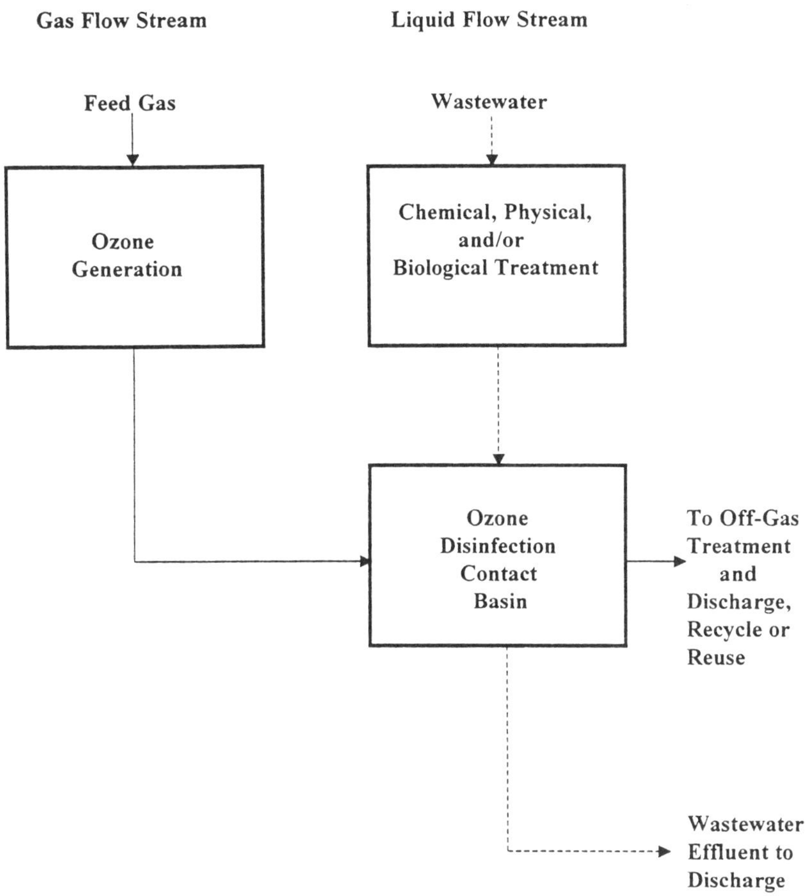

Figure 8.2 Ozone disinfection process gas and liquid flow diagram. *Source:* USEPA (1986), p. 108.

the receiving water. Any residual ozone in the wastewater is reacted or is reverted back to oxygen.

8.6.1 FEED-GAS FLOW

USEPA (1986) points out that ozone disinfection processes are typically distinguished by the type of feed-gas used. The most common types are air-fed and oxygen-fed. Oxygen recycle systems have been used on some occasions. (See Figure 8.3 for a diagram showing the components of these processes.) The air-fed system is most common in plants where oxygen is not available. Oxygen-fed systems are typically used in conjunction with an oxygen-activated sludge treatment system, where the unused oxygen from the ozone disinfection system is used in the biological treatment process.

For the electric discharge ozone generators, the quality of the feed-gas is critically important. It must be oil-free, particle-free, and dry. To remove moisture and particulates (and oil, if present), the gas to the air-fed (and oxygen recycle) systems must be pretreated.

Power requirements and the ozone generation equipment are about 50% lower for an oxygen-fed system than for an air-fed system, because approximately twice as much ozone is produced with high-purity oxygen at a given input of power to the generator. This lower cost of producing ozone is often offset, however, by a higher cost of obtaining high-purity oxygen to feed the generator. A beneficial economic trade-off occurs, however, whenever the oxygen can also be used in the biological system.

In all the feed-gas systems (see Figure 8.3), the ozone disinfection contacting units are similar. In the actual operation of an ozonation contact basin, some disinfection action occurs through direct contact of the microorganism with the ozone in the gaseous phase; however, "effective" disinfection appears to exist only when residual oxidants or an ozone residual is present. Note that to obtain residual oxidants or residual ozone, a sufficient amount of ozone must be transferred to the waters.

8.6.2 WASTEWATER FLOW SCHEMES

The USEPA (1986) provided several wastewater treatment schemes used prior to ozone disinfection that have been evaluated by various researchers (Figure 8.4). Based on various research modeling, the data gathered indicates

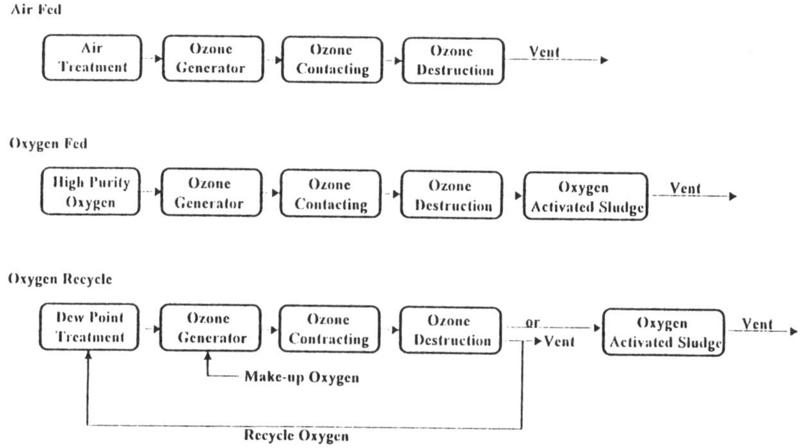

Figure 8.3 Diagrams showing feed-gas flow of typical ozone disinfection processes. *Source:* USEPA (1986), p. 108.

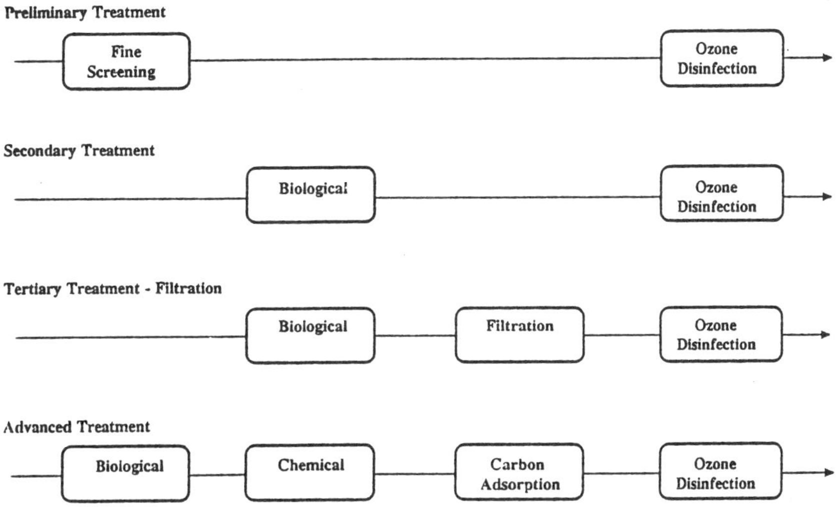

Figure 8.4 Example treatment schemes using ozone disinfection. *Source:* USEPA (1986), p. 110.

that there is no technical basis for excluding the use of ozone following any treatment scheme shown in Figure 8.4. However, depending on the type of wastewater treated and/or the effluent disinfection requirement, the wastewater treatment scheme may be an important economic consideration. An example of an ozone disinfection flow diagram is shown in Figure 8.5.

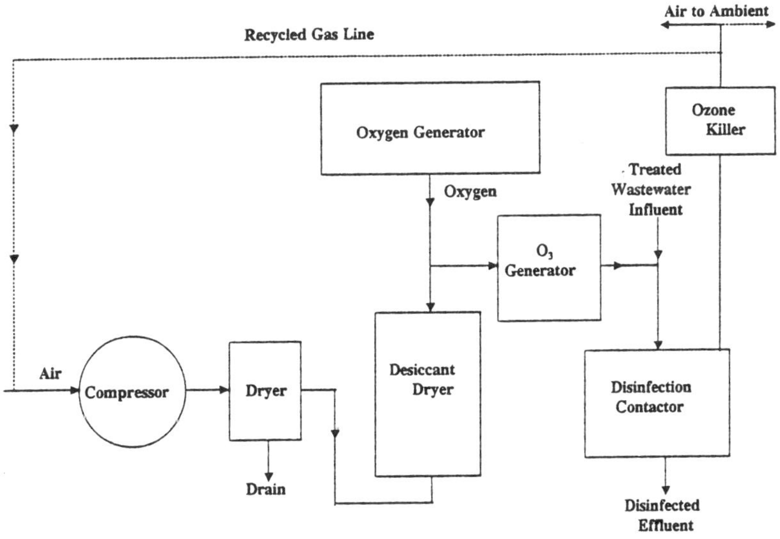

Figure 8.5 Ozone disinfection flow diagram. *Source:* Adaptation from G. C. White, p. 937, 1986.

8.7 OZONE: SAFETY CONSIDERATIONS

Like chlorine, ozone is a toxic gas and can cause severe illness and death if inhaled in sufficient quantity. Ozone has some advantages over chlorine use, however. Ozone is generated on-site, thus eliminating transportation hazards. Additionally, the generation system can be shut down if an ozone leak develops. Another safety advantage is the physical characteristic of ozone that allows it to be detected by odor at concentrations much lower than harmful levels. However, two areas of particular concern must be considered regarding the ozone operator's personal protection. Ozone process equipment makes "noise" (defined as unwanted sound at levels above OSHA action level 85 dBA and safe limits, i.e., >90 dBA). Protection against electrical hazards should be incorporated into the design and operation of an ozone disinfection system.

8.8 OZONE: THE DISCUSSION

Tuesday morning the DST reconvened and put together their list of findings and recommendations on ozone.

Findings:

(1) Ozone is a strong oxidizing gas that reacts with many organic molecules.
(2) It is produced (on-site) when oxygen molecules separate, collide with other oxygen atoms, and form a molecule consisting of three oxygen atoms.
(3) For high-quality effluents, ozone is a very effective disinfectant.
(4) Current regulations for domestic treatment systems limit use of ozonation to filtered effluents, unless the system's effectiveness can be demonstrated prior to installation.
(5) For ozonation of wastewater, the facility must have the capability of generating pure oxygen along with an ozone generator.
(6) A contact tank with ≥10-minute contact time at design average flow is required.
(7) Off-gas monitoring for process control is also required. In addition, safety equipment capable of monitoring ozone in the atmosphere and a ventilation system to prevent ozone levels exceeding 0.1 ppm are required.
(8) The actual operation of the ozonation process consists of monitoring and adjusting the ozone generator and the control system to maintain the required ozone concentration in the off-gas. The process must also be evaluated periodically by using biological testing to assess its effectiveness.

At this point in the proceedings, the DST felt that it had enough information on ozone to fit the data into their standard matrix (see Table 8.1).

Recommendations: Though ozone is a proven disinfectant, the jury is still out on the use of ozone in disinfecting wastewater. This is evidenced by the 40+ facilities that have incorporated ozone disinfection in their wastewater treatment process; later, almost half this number substituted some other alternative disinfection process than ozonation. From the data contained in the matrix, we see that ozone is not a viable disinfection alternative for use at Rachel's Creek (or anywhere else at the Authority) for the following reasons.

In addition to the fact that ozonation is a process that is still being studied for use in wastewater treatment, consider some of the data listed in the matrix (Table 8.1). In the first place, ozonation is a complex process; we have no experience with ozonation at the Authority. Second, ozonation does not produce a persistent residual (chlorine must be used to augment the ozonation disinfection process); instead of doing away with elemental chlorine, we would still have to use it at varying amounts for this particular process. Finally, the ozone factor of most concern to the DST (and the Authority) is

TABLE 8.1. Matrix for Determining the Applicability of Alternative Disinfection Techniques.

Alternative Disinfection Technique (e.g., Cl_2, BrCl, and O_3)	
Consideration	Ozone
Size of plant	Medium to large
Applicable level of treatment prior to disinfection	Secondary
Equipment reliability	Fair to good
Process control	Developing
Relative complexity of technology	Complex
Safety concerns—transportation on-site	No, moderate
Bactericidal	Good
Virucidal	Good
Fish toxicity	None expected
Hazardous by-products	None expected
Persistent residual	None
Contact time	Moderate
Contributes D.O.	Yes
Reacts with ammonia	Yes (high pH only)
Color removal	Yes
Increased dissolved solids	No
pH dependent	Slight (high pH)
O & M sensitive	High
Corrosive	Yes
Covered by PSM/RMP	Yes (PSM threshold quantity 100 lbs.)

the PSM threshold limit of 100 lb. Instead of substituting chlorine for some other alternative because of regulatory pressure, the ozone-substitution-for-chlorine scenario would be nothing more than swapping one covered chemical for another.

8.9 OZONE: THE BOTTOM LINE

Rain penetrated the darkness and spattered lightly against her condominium's windows. In the distance, a fog horn sounded its eerie solitary refrain. The streetlight to her right was dimly visible, its faint halo softly apparent in the darkness, fog, and rain. She stood at the window, watching the faint streaks of rain falling past the light. Solitary? No, just lost in thought. Thoughts about ozone? Not really; ozone was ancient history. The DST had finished its work on ozone earlier in the week and was now studying UV in preparation for Monday's meeting.

What was she thinking about? What absorbed her thoughts to the point that she was oblivious to everything else? Nancy Jo was going over that UNICEF article on solar disinfection of drinking water. She was recounting the steps.

"In order to save time and effort, it is highly desirable for a housewife to make her own arrangements to carry out the routine disinfection operation regularly once a day, or once every other day. For this reason, a housewife should ensure enough containers that would hold the desired quantity of drinking water estimated by her to meet the needs of the family for one or two days." Her mind recreated the procedure. Meanwhile, on this particular night, a torrent of fairly well disinfected water (disregarding its acid content) continued to strike her windows.

The survey forms were still rolling in; total number of respondents to date: 163 and still counting.

8.10 REFERENCES

Bell, J. B. and Smith, D. W. Wastewater Disinfection: Evaluation of Significant Factors. *Environ. Technol. Lett.*, 3, 319, 1982.

Caverson, et al. Ozone Disinfection of Primary Effluent Using a Stirred Tank Reactor. *Can. J. Civ. Eng.*, 13, 510, 1986.

Given, P. W. and Smith, D. W. Disinfection of Dilute, Low Temperature Wastewater Using Ozone. *Ozone Sci. Eng.*, 1, 91, 1979.

Hammer, M. J. and Hammer, M. J., Jr. *Water and Wastewater Technology* (3rd ed.). Englewood Cliffs, NJ: Prentice-Hall, 1996.

Malkin, M. and Fumento, M. *Rachel's Folly: The End of Chlorine.* Washington, D.C.: Competitive Enterprise Institute (no date).

McGhee, T. J. *Water Supply and Sewerage* (6th ed.). New York: McGraw-Hill, 1991.

Rakness, K. L., et al. Ozone Contactor Sizing Based on Demand, Decay and Equipment Criteria. In *IOA, Pan American Committee Meeting. Int. Ozone Assoc.,* Richmond, Virginia, 1994.

Rosen, H. M. Ozone Wastewater Disinfection: State-of-the-Art. In *Forum on Ozone Disinfection.* E.G. Fochtman et al. (Ed.), Inter. Ozone Inst., Chicago, Illinois, 1976, 36.

UNICEF, *Solar Disinfection of Drinking Water and Oral Rehydration Solutions.* American University of Beirut (1984).

Venosa, A. D., et al. Disinfection of Filtered and Unfiltered Secondary Effluent in Two Ozone Contactors. *Environ. Int.,* 4, 299, 1980.

USEPA. *Design Manual: Municipal Wastewater Disinfection*, 1986.

CHAPTER 9

UV Disinfection

Even before Mary Mallon (a.k.a. Typhoid Mary) was "cooking up" her daily food preparations (she was an American cook in the late 1800s and early 1900s) and passing on typhoid to her unsuspecting victims, people had suspected a relationship between microorganisms and disease. As a matter of historical record, even before the discovery of waterborne, disease-causing microorganisms, people suspected a relationship between water and the spread of disease. The quest for the truth about disease and disease-causing microorganisms began almost 2,600 years ago. This was the time frame when Hippocrates, the father of medicine, suspected that "different" waters caused several different diseases. It took several more centuries before Leeuwenhoek invented the microscope in 1675. Leeuwenhoek's microscope, with several later refinements, opened up the microscopic world. Giardia lamblia *was the first microorganism studied and described by Leeuwenhoek. Eventually, in the nineteenth century, other great men of science such as Koch and Pasteur disproved the ancient theory of poisonous vapors arising from decaying filth as the cause of disease; instead, they developed the germ theory. (F. R. Spellman, p. 118, 1997)*

9.1 SHEDDING SOME LIGHT ON THE SUBJECT

NANCY Jo couldn't understand why this single train of thought seemed to possess her. "At the end of the sunlight exposure period, a housewife could then transfer indoors the whole set of containers for use. To avoid recontamination, the already disinfected water should preferably be kept in the same containers used in the solar exposure operation. However, if there is a shortage of small containers, then the disinfected water could be transferred from each exposed container to a clean large container reserved for bulk storage of processed water."

"Once a set of emptied containers becomes available after usage, the refilling and exposure procedures are repeated. If the containers are maintained in a good state of cleanliness, then there would be no reason for having to clean them repeatedly each time they are to be re-used" (UNICEF, p. 1, 1984).

The UNICEF account of solar disinfection of drinking water haunted her each time the steps of the procedure recommended by UNICEF for disinfecting drinking water in developing nations ran through her mind—developing nations where 400 children under 5 years old die every hour from diarrheal diseases, including cholera and typhoid, diseases transmitted by contaminated drinking water (Valenti, 1997).

Eventually, though, Nancy Jo realized what she found so disturbing about the process. She put herself in the "housewife's" position, trying to imagine going through this ongoing, daily, never-ending, back-breaking routine of disinfecting the family's drinking water supply. Nancy Jo, of course, had never had to think about her water supply. She had a hard time trying to imagine all the steps it must entail for a household in a rural area with no safe water supply—couldn't fathom having to perform such a basic and necessary function. She had never had to worry about disinfecting her own drinking water supply; that was something that someone else did, that someone else thought about, that someone else worried about (hopefully).

Reading the UNICEF account haunted her because it had opened her—twenty-five-year-old Ph.D. in Environmental Science, specialty water pollution control technology—eyes to the fact that for many of us, reaching for a clean drinking glass, placing it under the tap, and filling it to the brim with cold, refreshing, clean, disinfected, safe water is no big deal. In America and Europe and a few other parts of the world, clean, disease-free drinking water is no concern, because it's available; not all of the world's inhabitants are so lucky. This was an eye-opener.

"We are so lucky, so very lucky, here in America," she told herself. But how much is luck? Too many elements to list were all factors in the infrastructure that provides most Americans with effective water treatment—good science, concerned government, adequate supply, good engineering, and money. Once she thought about it, Nancy Jo understood.

9.2 EARLY START

On Monday, Nancy Jo had arrived at her office before 6:00 A.M. In the 2 hours before the DST would meet, Nancy Jo completed some serious reading on the last disinfection alternative to be discussed: ultraviolet (UV) radiation or disinfection (see Figure 9.1).

Note: Although used interchangeably with radiation, irradiation is the proper term, which means to send forth rays; radiate. We use the term UV disinfection.

Nancy Jo already knew something about UV disinfection. However, she

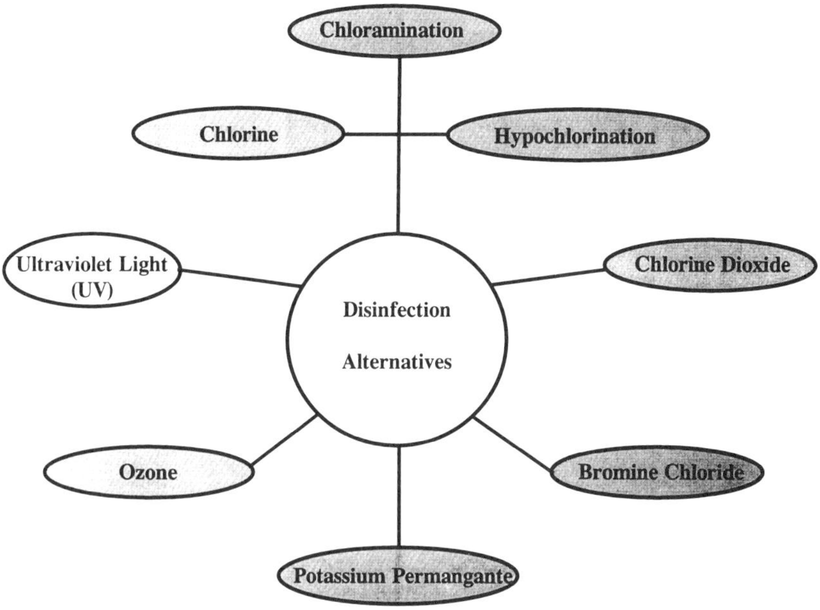

Figure 9.1 Ultraviolet light alternative.

felt she needed to learn much more. During the week, while she read everything and anything she could find on the subject, she had made a series of notes for today's DST session. During the 2-hour period prior to the DST session, she looked over her notes, rereading some thoroughly, including one she had made from the Water Environment Research Foundation's (WERF) *Comparison of UV Irradiation to Chlorination: Guidance for Achieving Optimal UV Performance* (1995). She read the WERF note again as food for thought:

"Wastewater disinfection has traditionally been accomplished using some form of chlorination. While an effective disinfectant, chlorine (and related compounds) has recently come under intense scrutiny because of regulatory and safety issues. In recent times, UV radiation has been used as an alternative for wastewater disinfection . . . Based on the many advantages of UV disinfection over dechlorination, it appears that the use of UV disinfection will continue to increase in the future. It is anticipated that as existing chlorine disinfection facilities reach their useful life, many will be replaced with UV disinfection facilities. Further, as newer UV technology is developed (e.g., medium pressure lamps and new ballasts) it is anticipated that capital and operation and maintenance costs will decrease, making UV disinfection even more cost competitive" (p. 1, 1995).

Then (just before the 8:00 meeting), she reread the UV parameter definitions she had listed earlier.

- *Water transmittance (UV demand)* The UV demand is similar to chlorine demand and is induced by chemical compounds that absorb UV radiation (proteins, phenols, humic material, lignin sulfonate, and iron compounds).
- *Turbidity and suspended solids* Suspended solids/turbidity can shadow (occlude) microorganisms, thus preventing the UV light from killing the microorganisms. As the level of suspended solids increases, the disinfection efficiency decreases.
- *Particle size* For similar levels of suspended solids, the larger the particle size, the lower the efficiency of UV disinfection.
- *Iron* Iron absorbs UV light and increases the rate of scaling/fouling of UV lamps.
- *Total dissolved solids and hardness* TDS and hardness can degrade system performance by scaling the quartz lamp sleeves. The scale decreases the UV intensity transmitted to the water, affecting the UV dosage.
- *Ultraviolet bank* A grouping of UV modules that spans the entire width and depth (of flow) of the reactor.
- *Ultraviolet module* A group of UV germicidal lamps of a specified arc length in a quartz or Teflon sleeve, sealed and supported in a single stainless steel or some other noncorrosive frame.
- *Ultraviolet radiation (UV)* Radiation that falls between visible light waves and x-rays. The longest UV waves have wavelengths slightly less than those of violet light (the limits of the human eye).
- *Ultraviolet radiation (UV) source* The low-pressure mercury arc lamp is the principal means of generating UV energy used for disinfection, at present. The mercury lamp is favored, because about 85% of the light output is monochromatic (having only one color) at a wavelength of 253.7 nm, which is within the optimum range (250 to 270 nm) for germicidal effects. The lamps are typically about 2.5 to 5.0 ft (0.75 to 1.5 m) in length, and about 0.6 to 0.8 in (15 to 20 mm) in diameter. To produce UV energy, the lamp, which contains mercury vapor, is charged by striking an electric arc. The energy generated by the excitation of the mercury vapor contained in the lamp results in the emission of UV light. Operationally, the lamps are either suspended outside of the liquid to be treated or submerged in the liquid. Where the lamps are submerged, the lamps are encased in quartz tubes to prevent cooling effects on the lamps (Metcalf and Eddy, 1991).

9.3 UV: BACKGROUND INFORMATION

Nancy Jo presented the following information to the DST.

Ultraviolet radiation or irradiation (UV) disinfection is a physical method that focuses on direct attack by ultraviolet light (at a wavelength of 254 nm) of the nucleic acids of bacteria, viruses, and other cellular organisms, thereby preventing cellular replication and ultimately causing death of the organism. The effectiveness of UV light as a bactericide and virucide has been well established.

Although ultraviolet disinfection was recognized as a method for achieving disinfection in the late nineteenth century, its application virtually disappeared with the evolution of chlorination technologies. However, in recent years, a resurgence for use in the wastewater field has occurred, largely as a consequence of concern for discharge of toxic chlorine residual. Even more recently, UV has gained more attention because of the tough new regulations on chlorine use imposed by both OSHA (PSM) and USEPA (RMP). Because of this relatively recent increased regulatory pressure, many facilities are actively engaged in substituting chlorine for other disinfection alternatives. UV technology itself has made many improvements, which now make UV an attractive disinfection alternative.

Ultraviolet light has very good germicidal qualities and is very effective in destroying microorganisms. It is used in hospitals, biological testing facilities, and many other similar locations. In wastewater treatment, the plant effluent is exposed to ultraviolet light of a specified wavelength and intensity for a specified contact period. The effectiveness of the process depends on:

- UV light intensity
- contact time
- wastewater quality (turbidity and TSS)

In the past, the Achilles' heel of UV for disinfecting wastewater has been turbidity problems. If the wastewater quality is poor, ultraviolet light is unable to penetrate the solids, and the effectiveness of the process decreases dramatically. For this reason, many states limit the use of UV disinfection to facilities that can reasonably be expected to produce an effluent containing $\leq$30 mg/L or less of BOD_5 and total suspended solids (TSS).

In the operation of a UV system, UV lamps must be readily available when replacements are required. The best lamps are those with a stated operating life of at least 7,500 hours and that do not produce significant amounts of ozone or hydrogen peroxide. The lamps must also meet technical specifications for intensity, output, and arc length. If the UV light tubes are submerged in the wastestream (see Figure 9.2), they must be placed inside quartz tubes, which protect the lights and make cleaning and replacement easier.

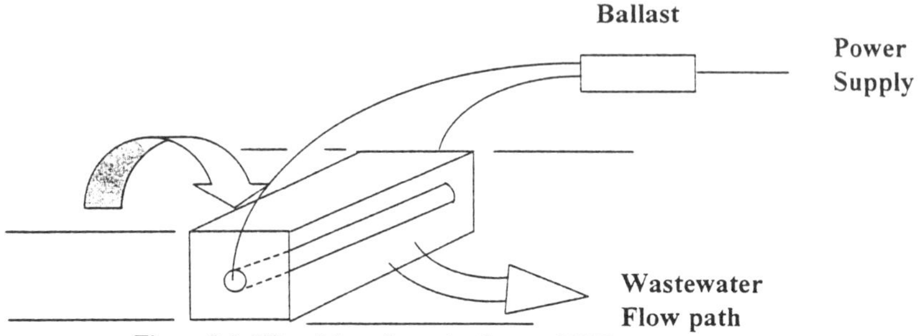

Figure 9.2 Ultraviolet schematic. *Source:* USEPA, p. 158, 1986.

In the past, contact tanks were required for use with UV disinfection. However, technological advances now make UV disinfection implementable in flow-through channels without the need for contact tanks. They may be designed with the banks of UV lights in a horizontal position either parallel or perpendicular to the flow or with banks of lights placed in a vertical position perpendicular to the flow.

Note: Contact tanks must provide a minimum of 10-second exposure time.

Turbidity problems have been the drawback with using UV in wastewater treatment; this is still the case. However, if turbidity is UV's Achilles' heel, then the need for increased maintenance (compared with other disinfection alternatives) has, in the past, been the toe of the same foot. Recent advances in technology have lessened this concern.

UV maintenance requires that the tubes be cleaned on a regular basis or as needed. Periodic acid washing is also required to remove chemical buildup.

In operating a UV disinfection system, routine monitoring is required to check on bulb burnout, buildup of solids on quartz tubes, and UV light intensity.

An important safety concern we need to take into consideration is that UV light is extremely hazardous to the eyes. Proper safety training and equipment would be essential. Workers must never enter areas where UV lights are in operation without proper eye protection and must never look directly into the ultraviolet light.

9.4 UV: DISCUSSION

After Nancy Jo completed her introductory presentation, the DST began discussing the advantages and disadvantages of UV disinfection as a possible disinfection alternative for use at Rachel's Creek Treatment Plant. The information on the record included:

- UV disinfection is an environmentally safe, nonchemical, physical process that produces no toxic side effects (WERF, 1995).

- UV radiation effectively destroys bacteria and viruses.
- As with ozone, a secondary disinfectant must be used to prevent regrowth of microorganisms and for other plant applications.
- The equipment is relatively easy to operate and maintain and is safe and simple for operators to use. It typically consists of multiple standard high-quality UV lamps, sealed within quartz tubes or sleeves. Wastewater flows around and past the quartz tubes and is thereby exposed to the UV radiation (see Figure 9.2).
- UV disinfection is able to achieve the required disinfection level in a few seconds, whereas chlorine requires 1/4 to 1/2 hour (WERF, 1995).
- The effectiveness of the UV system is affected by a number of factors, including potential fouling of the quartz sleeves. Therefore, maintenance of a UV system is required to keep the sleeves clean. Lamps will need periodic replacement.
- UV disinfection creates no increase in total dissolved solids (TDS). Chlorination and dechlorination do.
- UV disinfection presents no concern of overdosing.
- UV disinfection is easy to control and has a consistent outcome.
- Because the effectiveness of UV disinfection is affected by turbidity problems (water quality problems), its applications are typically limited to secondary treated wastewaters. Water quality parameters often dictate whether UV disinfection is an effective disinfection alternative.
- UV dosage affects UV disinfection effectiveness. The UV dosage can be controlled by varying the number of lamps and the hydraulic detention time around the lamps.
- UV disinfection is a good alternative to chlorinating.
- George Tchobanglous, Professor Emeritus of Civil and Environmental Engineering at the University of California, Davis, in an interview with Valenti (1997) stated: "The main advantage UV has over standard disinfection techniques is that the light-based system eliminates the transport and use of chlorine." Even though the water is dechlorinated by the addition of other chemical compounds such as sulfur dioxide, residues of these toxic compounds remain in the water, which is a matter of increasing concern. There are no residuals left by UV-light systems, whose effectiveness has been improved with the development of more intense ultraviolet lamps. Now, one lamp can do the work of 20.
- With UV disinfection, avoiding costly RMP requirements is possible.

At this point in the discussion, the DST incorporated the information they had gathered into their standard matrix (Table 9.1).

TABLE 9.1. Matrix for Determining the Applicability of Alternative Disinfection Techniques.

Alternative Disinfection Technique (e.g., Cl_2, BrCl, and O_3)	
Consideration	UV Disinfection
Size of plant	Small to medium
Applicable level of treatment prior to disinfection	Secondary
Equipment reliability	Fair to good
Process control	Developing
Relative complexity of technology	Simple to moderate
Safety concerns—transportation on-site	No, minimal
Bactericidal	Good
Virucidal	Good
Fish toxicity	Nontoxic
Hazardous by-products	No
Persistent residual	None
Contact time	Short
Contributes D.O.	No
Reacts with ammonia	No
Color removal	No
Increased dissolved solids	No
pH dependent	No
O & M sensitive	Moderate
Corrosive	No
Covered by PSM/RMP	No

9.5 AT THE CROSSROADS

For a short time, they sat speechless. After what they had heard and read about UV disinfection and after they had reviewed the data they plugged into their matrix, they all understood that they were at a crossroads. Why? Because initially, the members of the DST thought that selecting the disinfection alternative to replace elemental chlorine would be somewhat easy to do; it would simply come down to one alternative and one alternative only: sodium hypochlorite with sodium bisulfite for dechlorination. But now they felt differently; they all felt (from the information presented) that UV disinfection might indeed be a viable disinfection alternative for Rachel's Creek.

However, even though Nancy Jo felt as the other DST members did about the efficacy of UV as a disinfection alternative, she also was sure of something else. The DST didn't know what she and they did not know about UV disinfection—UV's suitability for use by the Authority, and especially for use at Rachel's Creek treatment plant.

Nancy Jo broke the silence. "Well, it is obvious to all of us, I am sure, that UV may be a viable alternative to elemental chlorine." All the members of the DST nodded their heads in agreement with this statement.

She continued. "What we need to do is to find out more about UV, to find out if in fact it can be used at Rachel's Creek in place of chlorine. At this point, two things are certain: (1) If we choose UV instead of elemental chlorine, we may not have to comply with RMP; and (2) if we choose UV to replace chlorine, we better be able to justify our choice. Remember, we cannot choose an alternative disinfection process because it "feels good." Instead, we must choose our alternative because of the facts, based on science and engineering. Frankly, from the information we have, I don't think we have enough justification to select UV as our primary choice, or enough justification to reject it." Again all DST members indicated their approval.

"What I recommend is that we adjourn for today and reconvene on Wednesday at the normal time. In the meantime, I have some specific research areas to assign everyone. Each of us, on an individual basis, needs to gather information on the UV alternative. We need to gather facts. At Wednesday's meeting, we need to take these facts and assimilate the information. In a sense, what we will be doing tomorrow is gathering information to develop a screening mechanism for determining the applicability of UV disinfection to our situation, and then we should be able to determine if we know enough or if we still don't know enough. Are we in agreement?"

The DST agreed with Nancy Jo's recommendation; she gave each member a specific research assignment and then adjourned the meeting.

9.6 UV SCREENING CRITERIA

Promptly at 8:00 Wednesday morning, the DST reconvened. Nancy Jo stood at the head of the conference table and began the session.

"Have you all been able to gather the data we need for today's session?" All of the DST members answered in the affirmative. Nancy Jo asked for a copy of each member's findings. Findings in hand, along with the data she had gathered, she had her assistant make a copy of the entire package for each DST member.

The DST spent the rest of the day digesting the data and information the team had gathered. By 5:00 that afternoon, the DST felt it had enough information, organized properly, to move on with their discussion and study. They decided to call it a day and reconvene Thursday morning at the regular time.

With DST's UV information neatly stacked in front of her, Nancy Jo began the discussion on Thursday at 8:00 A.M.

We have identified screening criteria to determine if Rachel's Creek Treatment Plant is suitable for UV disinfection. Keep in mind that the criteria we are about to list on the flip chart is approximate and are set to evaluate UV disinfection feasibility. Actual criteria will depend on testing of the wastestream. These data are provided from previous pilot studies on expected new sources of influent and from actual data taken from the existing wastewater influent presently entering Rufus' Crag POTW, which, as you all know, will be partially diverted to Rachel's Creek when it is completed.

The screening criteria to be used in the screening process for Rachel's Creek includes:

- *Effluent permit requirements* the level of disinfection and water parameters required by NPDES permit.
- *Total Suspended Solids* (forecasted value)
- *Turbidity* (forecasted value)
- *Filter requirement* Is a filter required prior to UV disinfection? If effluent quality dictates, then a filter may be required prior to UV disinfection. A pump station would have to be installed to provide additional hydraulic load.
- *Chlorine use* Will expected chlorine use in other Rachel's Creek processes (e.g., odor control, foam control, and thickener chlorination) separate from effluent disinfection trigger the RMP compliance requirements? If the chlorine use in other Rachel's Creek processes triggers the RMP, a scrubber would have to be built. Building a scrubber, complying with other RMP requirements and costs, and various codes, and installing UV disinfection may be cost-prohibitive.
- *Scrubber option* Is a scrubber included in the engineering specifications for the preliminary plans? If so, UV disinfection may be viable, even though projected chlorine use in other Rachel's Creek processes triggers the RMP requirements.
- *Ease of construction* Will new modifications be required to the preliminary plans and drawings to incorporate the UV disinfection alternative?
- *Use of iron salts* Use of iron in wastewater treatment processes makes UV disinfection less certain and increases the potential for problems from scaling and fouling of UV lamps.
- *Receiving water* If the toxicity of chlorine to sensitive receiving waters is a concern, UV is a desirable alternative.

9.6.1 PRELIMINARY SCREENING RESULTS

From Table 9.2's information on initial screening, the following criteria obviously had no discernible impact on the selection of the UV alternative:

- effluent permit requirements

TABLE 9.2a. Effluent Permit Requirements.

Projected Monthly Average					
TSS/mg/L	BOD mg/L	Coliform N/CML	TSS mg/L Projected Average	Turbidity NTUs*	Is Filter Required?
30	30	200	8	40	No

*NTU = nephelometric turbidity units used to measure turbidity.

TABLE 9.2b. Preliminary Screening Criteria for UV Disinfection.

Rachel's Creek POTW			
Do Other Cl_2 Uses Trigger RMP?	Does Projected Scrubber Meet RMP Requirements?	Ease of Construction	Use of Iron Salts
Yes	No	Yes	Yes

TABLE 9.2c. Preliminary Screening Criteria for UV Disinfection.

Rachel's Creek POTW	
Receiving Water Class	II

- filter requirement
- receiving water

The effluent permit requirements are typical (standard) and (in this case) have no bearing on the selection of any of the disinfection alternatives, including UV. Filters are not essential for the level of performance required at Rachel's Creek (a secondary plant: fecal coliform = 200 MPN/100 mL). Additionally, preliminary design specifications do not call for a filter or filters in the Rachel's Creek project. The plant is not presently designed to provide sufficient head to accommodate filters. Rachel's Creek will discharge to Class II water. Results of the remaining criteria (secondary criteria) are summarized below and shown in Table 9.3.

TABLE 9.3. Secondary Screening for UV Disinfection.

Cl_2 Use* (Other Than Disinfection) lb/day	Proposed Scrubber Meets RMP Requirements?	Iron Salt Use	Turbidity Projected NTUs Average	TSS (mg/L)
6208	No	Secondary	4	9

*Cl_2 use (other than disinfection) includes odor control, foam control, and thickener chlorine.

9.6.2 SECONDARY SCREENING RESULTS

Using the data contained in Tables 9.2 and 9.3, the DST eliminated UV disinfection from further consideration. The exact reasoning involved (the elimination factors) in this process is documented below.

UV Elimination Factors:

- *Other chlorine uses and scrubber option* UV disinfection becomes more economical if other chlorine demands (e.g., odor control, foam control, RAS, thickener disinfection) are low enough to avoid a scrubber installation and other RMP requirements. Table 3 shows the projected loadings (6,208 lb/day) from other chlorine uses for Rachel's Creek. Obviously, Rachel's Creek requires more than 2,500 pounds per day of chlorine for other uses. Because the prospective plant manager for Rachel's Creek stated that she will want to have the flexibility of having at least two chlorine containers on-line, with two more in back up at all times (a total of 10,000 lb of chlorine), this would exceed the RMP limit of 2,500 lb of on-line chlorine storage. Because Rachel's Creek will require more than 2,500 lb/day of chlorine for other uses, this constitutes justification for elimination of UV disinfection from further consideration.
- *Iron salts* The potential for accelerated scaling/fouling of the UV lamps increases as the iron addition location moves closer to the UV system. We project that Rachel's Creek will add iron in the secondary clarifiers. Thus, UV is eliminated from further consideration at Rachel's Creek, because of its potential for increased scaling and fouling of UV lamps.
- *Turbidity and TSS* Turbidity at (4 NTUs) and TSS at (8 mg/L) were conservatively estimated for Rachel's Creek. Although these values are not inordinately high (relatively speaking), they are high enough to cause concern. Thus, the use of UV as a disinfection agent at Rachel's Creek is eliminated from further consideration, because of potentially high turbidity and TSS, which could interfere with the disinfection function of the UV system.

9.7 THE BOTTOM LINE

At this point in the proceedings the members of the DST were comfortable with their findings. Comfortable, but not finished with the proceedings and the process.

Basically, what they had accomplished to date was the elimination of six of the eight disinfection alternatives. Although they felt that they had prepared adequate documentation to justify their decisions to date, the two remaining alternatives (elemental chlorine and sodium hypochlorite) had not been definitively compared and analyzed one-on-one. This remained to be accomplished. In addition, they still had to state emphatically which of the two alternatives was best suited for use at Rachel's Creek. The DST understood that stating an opinion is relatively easy; backing the opinion up with something concrete (e.g., data) is a different matter.

Nancy Jo decided that the DST should call it a day. However, before they adjourned, she informed the team members that their next meeting would be on Monday. At Monday's meeting, they would determine the pros and cons of using elemental chlorine or sodium hypochlorite at Rachel's Creek. After doing so, the DST would finalize its recommendation to the GM, which Nancy Jo would deliver and explain.

As they departed from the conference room, Nancy Jo could still hear the GM's words echoing in her memory. "You will be hard-pressed to change my mind about using anything but chlorine for disinfecting wastewater. You will have to put forward a strong recommendation and convincing evidence of the need to use 'some' technology other than elemental chlorine before I will be convinced."

The survey forms were still coming in; total number of respondents to date: 164 and still counting, but not for long.

9.8 REFERENCES

Metcalf and Eddy. *Wastewater Engineering: Treatment, Disposal, Reuse*. New York: McGraw-Hill Inc., 1991.

Spellman, F. R. *Microbiology For Water/Wastewater Operators*. Lancaster, PA: Technomic Publishing Company, Inc., p. 118, 1997.

UNICEF. *The Solar Disinfection of Drinking Water and Oral Rehydration Solutions*. American University of Beirut, 1984.

USEPA. *Design Manual: Municipal Wastewater Disinfection*, 1986.

Valenti, M. *From Municipal Wastewater to Spent Metalworking Fluids, Ultraviolet-Lighting Systems Offer Effective Disinfection*. American Society of Mechanical Engineers (ASME), 1997.

WERF. *Comparison of UV Irradiation to Chlorination: Guidance for Achieving Optimal UV Performance*, 1995.

CHAPTER 10

The Disinfection Alternative for Rachel's Creek

An excursion to the local stream can be a relaxing and enjoyable undertaking. On the other hand, when you arrive at the local stream, spread your blanket on the streambank and then look out upon the stream's flowing mass only to discover a parade of waste and discarded rubble bobbing along the stream's course and cluttering the adjacent shoreline and downstream areas, any feeling of relaxation or enjoyment is quickly extinguished. Further, the sickening sensation the observer feels is not lessened, but made worse as he gains closer scrutiny of the putrid flow. He easily recognizes the rainbow-colored shimmer of an oil slick, interrupted here and there by dead fish and floating refuse, and the slimy fungal growth that prevails. At the same time, the observer's sense of smell is alerted to the noxious conditions. Along with the fouled water and the stench of rot-filled air, the observer notices the ultimate insult and tragedy: The signs warn, "DANGER—NO SWIMMING or FISHING." The observer soon realizes that the stream before him is not a stream at all; it is little more than an unsightly drainage ditch. The observer has discovered what ecologists have known and warned about for years. That is, contrary to popular belief, rivers and streams do not have an infinite capacity for pollution. (F. R. Spellman, p. 65, 1996)

10.1 FORGING A DECISION

THE DST had convened as scheduled on Monday and had been hard at work until they reached their final decision Thursday afternoon. They spent Friday helping Nancy Jo put together the final report for presentation to the GM, which she had scheduled for Monday morning at 10:00 A.M.

The first 2 hours of Nancy Jo's presentation had gone well enough. She had placed all of the DST's pertinent information and findings into a Power-Point presentation. This presentation contained a summary of the materials the DST had waded through and sorted out in making their selection of sodium hypochlorite as the disinfection alternative of choice for Rachel's Creek Treatment Plant.

When lunch time approached, the GM told Nancy Jo that they would "lunch-in," so that they could continue on with the discussion. Nancy Jo didn't mind because she rarely went to lunch at all.

During lunch (while the GM ate), Nancy Jo continued her presentation. The information presented in the following is a record of what transpired over the next two hours.

10.2 STATING THE CASE

Using the USEPA's recommended procedure, the DST compared chlorine/sulfur dioxide and sodium hypochlorite/sodium bisulfite from the standpoint of both technical factors and feasibility considerations. The considerations are listed as follows:

- flexibility
- reliability
- complexity
- effectiveness
- pilot studies

For these considerations, the DST found virtually no difference between chlorine and sodium hypochlorite. However, we did find two unlisted and important considerations, where a considerable difference between the two disinfection alternatives does exist. These are:

- coverage by RMP
- costs

For coverage by RMP, our research has confirmed for us that chlorine use in the water/wastewater industries (and other industries) is a target for the USEPA. They have painted a bull's-eye on each container of chlorine, and the ammunition they are using is RMP.

Who knows what their real motivation is? Chlorine has been used in industries throughout the world reasonably safely and effectively, with no recorded Bhopals, Chernobyls, or Exxon Valdes', so the motivation for their "chlorine killer" regulation is anyone's guess. One thing is certain, though, water and wastewater industries throughout the United States have felt the heat, have gotten the message, have seen the light in regards to the USEPA's attack on chlorine usage and the chlorine user. When you get right down to it, it's the same old story, the same old regulatory modus operandi: If you can't stop an operation, such as the manufacture and distribution of a product, regulate it to death, and that is the plight of chlorine. On June 21, 1999 (when the requirements of RMP kick in), chlorine will die a slow death.

So, the question has become, "Does the Authority comply with USEPA's RMP requirements (the chlorine killer) or do we switch to something else?"

This leads to more questions. "If we decide to switch, what do we switch to?" The DST decided sodium hypochlorite is the answer (at least at the present time; you never know when the regulators will "kill" sodium hypochlorite).

The General Manager asked, "How do you know that water/wastewater industries have 'seen the light on chlorine,' as you have stated?"

Now that her trap had been set, sprung, and the victim captured, she proceeded with her presentation.

We know this because we conducted a survey throughout the country of 250 POTWs, so we would be able to make a determination of what they are doing in response to RMP requirements. (She handed the GM a copy of the survey results. See Table 10.1.)

Note: The DST had attached a list of each agency that responded, facility size, and a comment related to present status. To maintain confidentiality, the list is not included here.

While the GM was digesting his lunch, he was also digesting the survey results. After finishing his review of the list, he stated, "You said something about costs . . . what's the deal?"

We are actually concerned with two sets of costs here. The first set has to do with staying with chlorine (and complying with RMP), and the other set of costs has to do with substituting chlorine with sodium hypochlorite.

TABLE 10.1. RMP Survey Summary.

Number of agencies surveyed	250
Number of agencies reporting	166 (66.4%)
Number of facilities	378
Number staying w/Cl*	140 (37%)
Number switched/ing**	117 (31%)
Number undecided†	79 (21%)
Number of others‡	42 (11%)

*Of the 140 plants staying with Cl_2 and/or SO_2 gas:

- 62 plants have or plan to install scrubbers (44%).
- 36 plants do not plan to install scrubbers (26%).
- 42 plants either made no comment on scrubbers or other (30%).

**Of the 117 plants that have switched or are switching to alternatives:

- 59 plants have gone or are going to NAOCl (50%).
- 32 plants have gone or are going to UV (27%).
- 26 plants are switching but did not identify their chosen method of disinfection (23%)

†Of the 79 plants that are undecided: 28 plants stated they were evaluating disinfectants, but not due to RMP, etc. (39%)

‡Of the 42 plants in the other category:

- 16 plants are using alternative disinfectants, but not due to RMP, etc. (39%).
- 13 plants are using Cl_2 or SO_2, either below RMP, or status unknown, etc. (29%).

The capital, operations and maintenance, and present worth cost estimates are shown in Table 10.2.

In addition to Table 10.2, Nancy Jo also presented the GM with an attachment of the details of the cost estimate. The GM reviewed Table 10.2 for a few minutes, and then said: "Bottom line, what is this going to cost our customers on their monthly bill, for example?"

Nancy Jo replied, "Our 1.5 million customer base will see an increase in their monthly bills of approximately \$0.011 above what it will cost to go with hypo versus to install the chlorine scrubbers and comply with RMP; on an annual basis, we are talking an approximate increase of \$0.13 for the chlorine alternative."

The GM sat there in silence for a moment, and then asked: "If we install sodium hypochlorite at Rachel's Creek, what about our other facilities that are already using chlorine? I mean, it just doesn't make sense to me to single out Rachel's Creek for hypochlorite and still use chlorine at our other water/wastewater facilities. If we substituted hypochlorite for chlorine at the other facilities, what would that cost us and our customers?"

Nancy Jo answered, "Well, I can give you a rough ballpark figure if you want it." She turned to the page of her notes containing the information the

TABLE 10.2. Capital, Operations and Maintenance, and Present Worth Cost Estimate for Rachel's Creek Treatment Plant.

Parameter	Containment Scrubber (Cl_2) Alternative	Sodium Hypochlorite/ Sodium Bisulfite Alternative
Capital costs		
Sitework	\$22,000	\$11,000
Building (Cl_2/NaOCl)	\$355,000	\$340,000
Dechlorination building	\$82,000	\$84,000
Scrubber building	\$312,000	Not applicable
Facility subtotal	\$771,000	\$435,000
General requirements	\$48,000	\$49,000
Allowance for undefined items	\$119,000	\$121,000
Engineering/administration	\$72,000	\$73,000
Total capital costs	\$1,010,000	\$678,000
Annual O & M costs		
PSM/RMP	\$14,000	Not applicable
Chemicals	\$85,000	\$157,000
Electricity	\$1,200	\$1,200
Total annual O & M costs	\$100,200	\$158,200
Annual O & M present worth	\$910,000	\$1,440,000
Total alternative costs	\$1,920,000	\$2,118,000

Total alt. costs = total capital costs + annual O & M present worth.

GM requested (she had anticipated his question on this subject, obviously). "To go to hypochlorite rather than chlorine, it will cost our customers a total monthly increase in rates of $0.42 per month above what it would cost to install chlorine scrubbers and comply with RMP, approximately $5.00 per annum."

The GM said, "Do you realize how sensitive our customer base is to a rate increase, any rate increase?"

"Absolutely," replied Nancy Jo.

The GM sat there a few minutes, thinking. Nancy Jo stared at the photograph of golfer Bobby Jones hanging on the wall above and behind the GM's head.

Finally, the GM said, "I want to ask you a question, Nancy Jo, a very simple question, . . . and I want a straightforward answer.

"Let's assume for this instance that you and not me were sitting in this chair; as General Manager, what would you do and why?"

Without hesitation Nancy Jo replied, "I would go with hypochlorite, not only at Rachel's Creek but at all of our plants."

The GM looked at her, then said, "Yes. But you didn't answer why. So why? Tell me why."

Nancy Jo looked the GM right in the eye, and stated, "It is quite simple, actually. I like to sleep at night."

The GM sat back in his high-back leather chair, placed his feet up on the corner of the desk, folded his hands behind his head and sighed.

"That will be all, Nancy Jo. I will let you know what I decide in a day or so. Thank you for your effort on this matter. . . . You did a good, thorough job for us."

Nancy Jo got up from the chair and left the GM's office. She went directly to her office and back to her work.

After Nancy Jo was gone, the GM sat at his desk for a while in the same pose, feet up on desk, hands folded behind his head, staring at the ceiling fan above him. On the surface of his mind, he was thinking about his golf swing and on how he could get rid of the slice he had recently developed.

A few minutes later he got up, grabbed his golf bag, and headed to the local driving range. On his way out the office door, he looked back at the neatly packaged report on his desk and paused for just a moment. "She really made a hole-in-one," he said to himself. "I have to give Dr. Nancy Jo Snow credit. It turns out we have something in common. We both like to sleep at night. Always was kind of partial toward hypochlorite anyway."

10.3 REFERENCE

Spellman, F. R. *Stream Ecology and Self-Purification.* Lancaster, PA: Technomic Publishing Company, Inc., 1996.

Index